PHLEBOTOMY FOR NURSES
AND NURSING PERSONNEL

PHLEBOTOMY FOR NURSES

AND NURSING PERSONNEL

WHAT EVERY NURSE AND NURSING ASSISTANT MUST KNOW ABOUT BLOOD SPECIMEN COLLECTION

Dennis J. Ernst MT(ASCP)

Director, Center for Phlebotomy Education, Inc.
Phlebotomy Instructor, University of Louisville School of Allied Health Sciences

Catherine Ernst, RN

Nursing Education Liaison, Center for Phlebotomy Education, Inc.

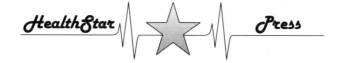

HealthStar Press

Publisher's Cataloging-in-Publication
(Provided by Quality Books, Inc.)

Ernst, Dennis J.
        Phlebotomy for nurses and nursing personnel /
by Dennis J. Ernst and Catherine Ernst. -- 1st ed.
        p. cm.
        Includes bibliographical references and index.
        LCCN: 00-103918
        ISBN: 0-9700588-9-6

        1. Phlebotomy--Handbooks, manuals, etc.
    I. Ernst, Catherine. II Title.

RB45.15.E76 2001   616.07'561
                                                QBI00-566

Printed in the United States of America on recycled paper

We dedicate this work to God, the ultimate author of our inspiration, our blessings, our lives.

TABLE OF CONTENTS

Preface
Acknowledgements

4. Alternative Sites, Blood Culture Collections, Phlebotomy Liability

5. Capillary Punctures, Pediatric Venipunctures

6. Specimen Handling and Storage

7. Managing Exposures to Bloodborne Pathogens

8. Practices and Products for Exposure Prevention

Appendices

Preface

The evolution of phlebotomy from a laboratory-based function to a nursing-based function impacts nurses in no small way. Although some institutions are blending several job classifications into one creating job titles such as "patient-care associate," "patient-care technician," or "clinical assistant," other institutions are handing phlebotomy duties directly to the nurse. It is not yet clear if this transition is permanent or a swing of a pendulum that will eventually return and restore phlebotomy to a laboratory-based function, but this much is clear: More and more nurses and their assistants are being asked to add blood collection skills to their growing list of responsibilities.

Arguments can be made ad nauseam on the negative consequence the transition of phlebotomy to a nursing-based function can have on the patient. But as patient advocates, we are obligated to tactfully articulate our concerns so that we might influence this transition in the best interests of the patient. At the same time, we are obligated to accept this role, and focus our efforts on minimizing its negative effects on the patient. It is for this latter duty that this book is written.

What this book is and isn't

This book attempts to present basic phlebotomy techniques with one goal: to teach techniques and principles that, when properly employed, protect the nurse from accidental needlesticks, protect the patient from injury, and result in the collection and transportation of high-quality specimens to the laboratory that are free of the multitude of variables collectors can introduce into specimens that alter results. That's it. No lengthy dissertations on esoteric phlebotomy procedures, no pedantic lectures on human anatomy or blood composition, and no tutorials on clinical laboratory science. You will not find an appendix of medical terminology, passages on the history of bloodletting, chapters on professionalism or how to draw blood on animals. This book is not intended to be a comprehensive, all-encompassing encyclopedia of blood collection. Such books already exist. (Healthcare professionals who are interested in a highly detailed text will find the 475-page *Phlebotomy Handbook* by Diana Garza and Kathleen Becan-McBride (Stamford, Conn, Appleton & Lange:1999) or *Phlebotomy Essentials* by Ruth E. McCall and Cathee M. Tankersley (Philadelphia, Penn, Lippincott-Raven:1998) to be excellent comprehensive texts on blood collection.)

Phlebotomy for Nurses and Nursing Personnel recognizes that nurses don't often have time to wade through large tomes written for entry-level phlebotomists in search of the core concepts of its subject. With today's nurse under the ever-increasing pressure to maintain current skills while juggling work, home, and parental responsibilities, any book that teaches a new procedure had better get to the point. That's what this book does.

Laboratories are sometimes viewed as mysterious entities to those who don't have the opportunity to see the inner workings of clinical testing facilities. To enhance readers' understanding of how the laboratory works, we've included unique "In the Lab" sidebars that illuminate some laboratory processes and how collection errors can impact the testing phase. We feel strongly, though, that anyone who collects blood specimens for clinical testing would benefit from spending one shift observing laboratory functions. It is reasonable to assume that investing in such firsthand experiences would result in higher quality specimens and fewer re-collections.

As expert witnesses in legal cases, we have seen the consequences of venipunctures improperly performed by those who are poorly trained and inadequately supervised. To help reinforce the concepts of proper technique and sound management practices, actual case studies are presented to give a human dimension to the consequences of poor technique. No other book on phlebotomy offers this kind of insight.

The NCCLS establishes the standand for blood specimen collection in the U. S. in document H3-A4, *Procedures for the Collection of Diagnostic Blood Specimen by Venipuncture*. Because this document is considered the standard in the industry, it is the framework of this text. All facilities should have a copy of this document for reference when drafting phlebotomy procedures and policies. Information for obtaining copies of this document and its companion video can be found in Appendix IV.

One of the greater challenges in healthcare today is to react to accidental needle-sticks with a calm, controlled approach, yet in a timely manner. That's why a great deal of research and time has gone into the chapter on exposure management. This chapter represents the most current information available at the time of this book's printing. We heartily encourage nurses and their assistants to make sure the exposure control plan in effect in their facility can respond to an exposure around the clock, 365 days a year. The plan within any facility should not rest solely on the shoulders of one person or one department. Every healthcare worker at risk of exposure has ownership in the plan and should take a personal interest in its functionality.

Because this text assumes an advanced understanding of nursing and a working knowledge of laboratory concepts, it has the luxury of being brief without compromising the essential. To make browsing easier, we have added page summaries in the margins that put the most essential concept of that page in a nutshell for a quick grasp of the page's content.

When writing about phlebotomy for a diverse nursing readership, choosing the proper term to address the reader is always a problem. Refer to the "nurse" and you leave out the nurse assistant who also draws blood; refer to "healthcare workers" and you sound too industrial. Therefore, begging the readers' understanding of this linguistic limitation, we ask permission to favor "healthcare professionals" as a general term in this context. We thank you for allowing us this liberty.

The authors

ACKNOWLEDGEMENTS

We could not have assembled this book without the many individuals who lent us their expertise and talents to make this text as accurate, useful and attractive as possible. We wish to thank Brian Jenkins of Digital Graphics and Cheryl Stewart for applying their creative talents to the cover design and Brian Jenkins (again!) for his graphic wizardry and file management expertise. We thank Ruth Carrico, RN and James Snyder, Ph.D., for their contributions to the exposure control and blood culture chapters respectively. We also wish to thank Dick Barnett, Vivian Bradbury of Sans Serif, Inc., Sheila Clover PBT(ASCP), Elizabeth Randall, BSN, RN, C, Sue Phelan MHS,MT(ASCP), and Rebecca Johnson, Ph.D.,RN for their invaluable advise on the text and all the product manufacturers who have provided us with illustrations.

Chapter 1

Phlebotomy as a Nursing Procedure: Managing the Risk

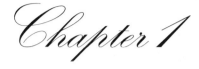

IDENTIFYING THE RISKS

The very nature of healthcare is to heal the sick and injured and to maintain the well-being of the healthy. This means exposure to body fluids and the disease-causing organisms they carry. Anyone who chooses a career in healthcare accepts that risk; but the choice has never been so great or the risk so manageable.

Phlebotomy does not expose nursing personnel to new risks, but it does expose them to greater risks than those they have grown accustomed to. One study shows phlebotomy to be the procedure most frequently associated with HIV exposure and that the risk of exposure is in part linked to the frequency with which healthcare professional perform blood drawing procedures.[1] Nursing personnel new to venous access procedures (eg, nursing assistants, patient care assistants, etc), however, are even more vulnerable to the risk, a fact that makes it even more urgent to establish comprehensive training, evaluation, and risk management practices.

> Of all healthcare professionals, nurses are at the highest risk for sustaining accidental needlesticks.

It has been estimated that healthcare workers suffer 1 million accidental needlesticks every year.[2,3] Hollow-bore needles, the kind used for collecting blood, account for 68.5 % of these.[3] The breakdown of needlesticks by profession is as follows*:[4]

Nurses	46%
Clinical laboratory workers	23%
Physicians	15%
Housekeepers/laundry workers	5%
Others	12%

*Total does not equal 100% due to rounding.

Even more alarming is that up to 92 % of accidental needle-stick injuries suffered by laboratory personnel go unreported.[3] Regardless of their function, all healthcare professionals must know that the necessary precautions cannot be ignored when drawing blood from a population stricken with injury, illness, and disease. Performing venous access procedures can expose the healthcare professional to at least 20 diseases.[5] Most of them are life-threatening, some of them deadly, and all of them preventable when the healthcare professional uses appropriate caution, technique, and equipment.

Needle Safety Legislation

The Occupational Safety and Health Administration's (OSHA) Bloodborne Pathogen Standard was implemented in 1992 to protect workers from acquiring bloodborne diseases. A directive was issued in 1999 to instruct inspectors to cite employers who do not utilize needleless systems and sharps with engineered protection.

In November of 2000, the Needlestick Safety and Prevention Act (HR5178) was signed into law to strengthen the enforcement of the OSHA directive. But OSHA guidelines alone will not protect all healthcare professionals. State, county, and municipal employees are exempt from federal OSHA regulations in states that do not have state OSHA departments (currently 29 states). In response to this shortfall, many of those states have passed needlestick legislation that applies the federal OSHA Bloodborne Pathogen Standard to all facilities. Additionally, federal lawmakers are considering legislation that removes the OSHA exemption from all state, county and municipal hospitals.

Readers who would like to view the text of the Needlestick Safety and Prevention Act are referred to http://www.Thomas.loc.gov and search for Bill Number HR5178. For updates on state legislative activity, visit the American Nurses Association's (ANA) Web site at http://www.ana.org or the International Health Care Worker Safety Center's Web site at http://www.med.Virginia.edu.

For a review of available products to protect healthcare workers who perform venipunctures, see Chapter 8, Practices and Products for Exposure Prevention.

Of the one million healthcare workers who suffer accidental needlesticks each year, it is estimated that 18 to 60 of them will contract HIV, 400-1000 will acquire hepatitis B and up to 9600 will become infected with the deadly hepatitis C virus.[6,7] These statistics present irrefutable evidence that phlebotomy technique must be taken seriously if healthcare professionals are to protect themselves from the devastating consequences of complacency, yet the responsibility is not theirs alone. Until employers demonstrate a commitment to protecting their staff through the exclusive use of safety needles or are forced to do so through legislation (see sidebar), the only protection healthcare professionals have against accidental needlesticks and the diseases they invite is a well-established technique acquired through comprehensive training and regular evaluation. Therefore, it is paramount for healthcare professionals and their employers to work together to assure that adequate safety policies are instituted, safety devices are made available, and safe practices are enforced.

> When assuming phlebotomy responsibilities, nursing personnel must be trained properly and must routinely employ sound safety practices to protect themselves from injury.

If the proper technique for collecting blood specimens is applied consistently, the risk of an accidental needlestick and patient injury can be significantly decreased. Nevertheless, allied healthcare professionals must strictly adhere to sound safety practices throughout their careers and resist the occasional temptation to deviate from safe practices. Likewise, those who evaluate skills must be continuously on guard for deviations from safe needle use and provide corrective guidance for those who demonstrate failure to comply.

Phlebotomy procedures are not new to nursing personnel who work in physicians' offices, home care, or in other outpatient capacities. However, more and more nursing departments in hospitals or long-term care facilities, who do not typically collect blood specimens are being asked to add phlebotomy to their list of responsibilities. (See box: *Phlebotomy as a Nursing Procedure*.) When those unfamiliar with the procedure are asked to acquire this additional skill with little input or training, the effects on the employees involved may include:

> ➢ Decreased morale
> ➢ Heightened concern for the patient's quality of care
> ➢ Increased risk of accidental needlesticks
> ➢ Anxiety of performing a new invasive procedure
> ➢ Sense of being overwhelmed by the demands of a new procedure.

The patient may suffer as well when the phlebotomist's needle is taken away from the specialist—whose skill has been honed by repetition—and given to someone for whom phlebotomy is far too occasional to be perfected. It stands to reason that if transitions are haphazardly implemented, patients will suffer. Reassigning phlebotomy responsibilities without providing adequate training can impact patients in many ways:

> Repeat punctures
> Traumatic punctures
> Patient misidentification
> Subcutaneous hemorrhages
> Temporary or permanent injuries
> Frequent and severe hematomas
> Erroneous results that lead to patient mismanagement.

Because these consequences for the patient and nursing personnel can be devastating, the decision to cross-train nurses to perform venipunctures, therefore, must be made with full knowledge of the potential outcomes. These risks can be effectively managed when facilities give a high priority to:

> Soliciting input from those healthcare professionals most affected by a phlebotomy transition
> Establishing a comprehensive phlebotomy training protocol
> Establishing and maintaining high standards of performance
> Drafting procedures that incorporate sound and safe phlebotomy techniques
> Implementing policies that protect the healthcare professional from accidental needlesticks
> Providing engineering controls that protect those performing phlebotomy procedures from injury.

A comprehensive training protocol that stresses safety and high standards of performance minimizes the risk of accidental needlesticks; those who are mindful of the impact such a transition will have on the morale of the staff maximizes the success of the transition.

MANAGING THE RISKS

Soliciting Input

When implementing change, managers who fail to integrate those most affected in the process risk alienating those whose input is critical to its success. Those most affected hold the key to a successful transition. Remember, asking healthcare professionals to take on phlebotomy responsibilities is asking them to perform a function that may be foreign to them, risky to their patients, and can have disastrous consequences if performed incorrectly. They fear for their patients; they fear for themselves. Resistance to change, therefore, is natural and should be anticipated. Managers who are insensitive to the effects that this change can have on their staff invite chaos, dissension and resistance while provoking a multitude of emotions.[8]

To ensure a successful transition of phlebotomy from a laboratory-based function to a nursing-based function, therefore, every attempt must be made to recruit the cooperation and input of those involved. It is prudent to begin with a sincere concern about the impact that the transition will have on the job performance of the staff members who will be affected. When approached with respect for their concerns, healthcare professionals may readily adopt the new role. Only when those affected understand the necessity for change will administrators and managers successfully recruit their cooperation and constructive input. Therefore, soliciting cooperation begins with an honest account of why it is necessary for those foreign to phlebotomy to learn the skill.

> Nursing personnel can demonstrate amazing adaptability to new responsibilities when administrators and managers give respect for their concerns over the impact multiskilling has on the quality of care they provide.

In hospitals, the need for administrators to restructure phlebotomy services can become necessary for a variety of reasons, not the least of which is economics. It is no secret that if hospitals don't function as a business, they don't function for long. However, administrators who communicate the market forces that bring about the need for the nursing staff to learn phlebotomy skills can at least make this transition understood, if not accepted. In addition, by providing adequate training, administrators infuse confidence and eliminate a significant apprehension, even fear of the procedure. For healthcare professionals, adjusting workloads to accommodate the added procedure can keep new responsibilities from becoming a burden.

Patients have no better defender of the quality of care that they are receiving than their immediate caregiver. The economics of healthcare often force a nursing staff to work under stressful and dangerous conditions and according to policies that actually interfere with the quality of care they want to provide. Managers and administrators do well to recruit the input of those affected by reassigned phlebotomy responsibilities. Engaging the players in every step of the process—conception, design, implementation, and monitoring—gives healthcare professionals a sense of ownership in the process rather than a feeling of victimization. Those who find themselves being forced to add one more procedure to their repertoire of skills

Phlebotomy as a Nursing Procedure:
An Historical Perspective

In the history of hospital-based healthcare, specimen collection began as a laboratory function. It made sense for those testing the blood to have control over all aspects of the specimen, including its collection. Then, in the 1970s, laboratories sensed a need to streamline their work flow and created blood collection specialists—*phlebotomists*—to collect and process specimens. Creating this position allowed the higher paid laboratory technologists to concentrate on the highly technical testing phase of clinical laboratory work. Because blood collection and its processing were their only responsibilities, phlebotomists perfected the technique and became highly skilled members of the healthcare team.

But as America's monstrously wasteful healthcare delivery machine lumbered through the 1980s and into the 1990s, healthcare providers were forced to take a hard look at the economics of their staffing patterns. To those who were responsible for keeping facilities solvent, it became increasingly obvious that employing individuals who have only one skill was an inefficient use of human resources. While it was true that phlebotomists allowed the higher paid laboratorians to concentrate on specimen analysis, those who weren't performing other laboratory functions in between venipunctures accumulated hours and hours of *downtime*, the elimination of which became the mantra of healthcare administrators, chief financial officers, and human resources directors industry-wide. Adding even more pressure to modify the role of the phlebotomist, patient satisfaction surveys began to show that the more employees patients encountered during their stay, the *less* satisfied they were with their care. This urged administrators to move phlebotomists to the bedside as caregivers capable of performing other direct patient care functions. Adding more appeal was the opportunity it presented to reduce their workforce (a perpetual objective) by combining positions. This restructuring concept heralded the beginning of the end for the one-skill, laboratory-based phlebotomist.

Gradually, the terms "cross-trained" and "multiskilled" echoed from the boardrooms and hallways to define those who could be trained to perform a multitude of formerly foreign functions without having a negative impact on patient care. Despite evidence to the contrary, the trend continues to make phlebotomy the responsibility of not only the newly designated "patient care associates" (or some similar variation), but to add blood collection procedures to the list of duties of the already-overburdened nurse.

In long-term care facilities the transition of phlebotomy to a nursing-based function has other origins. Reference laboratories are under increasing pressure to eliminate their phlebotomy services to their clients. The practice of providing free phlebotomy services in exchange for a facility's agreement to use their labs for reference work is now illegal in many cases. The Prospective Payment System enacted by Medicare makes it difficult for reference labs to provide this service even for a fee. Therefore, facilities for the aged are being forced to make other arrangements to have their residents' specimens collected. For most, the logical solution is to train their employees to collect the specimens themselves. Unfortunately, many facilities don't have the resources to train their staff to perform phlebotomy properly.

The industry continues to debate the wisdom of these transitions in theory and in practice.

will do well to become part of the process and interject constructive suggestions for implementation strategies and alternatives. Should phlebotomy become an inevitable addition to their responsibilities, healthcare professionals can work to minimize the negative effects that a cross-training strategy can bring to patients by learning the intricacies of the technique as they would any other procedure. At the same time, working to effect change can protect the patient and the healthcare employee from the negative impacts of healthcare economics.

Comprehensive Phlebotomy Training

Because phlebotomy seems deceptively simple, nurses and allied healthcare professionals are being asked to accept that the procedure requires little or no formal training. The result: missed veins, erroneous results, accidental needlesticks, acquired diseases, injured patients, and lawsuits. For nurses, the tendency is to equate phlebotomy with starting an IV. The difference, however, is profound. To assume that someone skilled at starting IVs can draw blood with little additional training is to put patient outcomes and careers at great risk. There are many nuances to collecting a blood specimen that, if not regularly employed, can result in injury and patient mismanagement. Risks include:

> Nursing personnel can work to minimize the negative effects that a cross-training strategy can bring to patients by perfecting new techniques as they would any other nursing function while effecting changes in administrative decisions that put patients at risk.

➢Incorrect diagnosis
➢Undermedicating a patient
➢Overmedicating a patient
➢Unnecessary increases in the length of stay
➢Premature discharge from the facility
➢Unnecessary transfusions
➢Untreated blood loss

➢Accidental arterial puncture
➢Neural involvement
➢Specimen misidentification
➢Specimen mishandling
➢Improper specimen storage
➢Accidental needlesticks.

These mistakes can result in a multitude of unnecessary outcomes including:

➢Internal hemorrhage
➢Septicemia
➢Unnecessary hospitalization
➢Stroke
➢Amputation
➢Myocardial infarction
➢Toxicity

➢Seizures
➢Insulin shock
➢Disabling injuries
➢HIV
➢Hepatitis
➢Death

With such sobering consequences from poorly performed venipunctures, it is imperative that healthcare professionals and their administrators apply the same importance to teaching proper phlebotomy technique as they would any other invasive procedure. Only through a comprehensive training program that teaches every aspect of phlebotomy to those who undertake the procedure can facilities and individuals guarantee their safety and the safety of their patients, the integrity of their specimens, and the preservation of the quality of care they strive to deliver.

There are no national standards that establish minimum training requirements to perform phlebotomy. The Joint Commission on Accreditation of Healthcare Organizations (JCAHO) requires that "Hospital's leaders define the qualifications and performance expectations for all staff positions," and "an orientation process provides initial job training and information and assess the staff's ability to fulfill specified responsibilities."* California has legislated a minimum training curriculum of 40 hours of classroom instruction, 40 hours of practical instruction and a minimum of 50 supervised punctures for all who draw blood except nurses, physicians, medical technologists, EMTs, and medical assistants who work in physician office labs. (See box: *Legislating Phlebotomy Certification* on page 11.) Although this requirement does not apply to nurses since it assumes nursing schools teach phlebotomy, it sets a standard for all healthcare professionals regardless of their discipline.

> **Phlebotomy is not "just like starting an IV."** Administrators who underestimate the importance of teaching this technique properly subject their patients to negative outcomes, including death.
>
> **Phlebotomy training should involve the perspectives of laboratory professionals.**

Following this precedent may seem unreasonably demanding to administrators or those who are involved in training and evaluating nursing personnel who perform venipunctures. However, if it can be proven that inadequate training contributed to a phlebotomy-related injury, there is little a facility can do to defend itself.

Because phlebotomy has historically been a laboratory function, there exists an expertise among laboratorians in the procedure. Therefore, any training program should be conducted in concert with a representative from the laboratory or a healthcare professional with a strong laboratory background to ensure that proper techniques are taught from a laboratory perspective.

Additionally, labs have a vested interest in the quality of the specimen. In fact, the Clinical Laboratory Improvement Amendments of 1988 (CLIA '88) deems that laboratories are ultimately responsible for the quality of the specimens it tests. Therefore, there is a legitimate need to infuse the laboratory perspective into any training program or in-service.

---

* ©Joint Commission: *CAMH: Comprehensive Accreditation Manual for Hospitals.* Oakbrook Terrace, IL: Joint Commission on Accreditation of Healthcare Organizations, 2000,HR-4. Reprinted with permission.

Case Study
A hospital in the Midwest hired a phlebotomist who had recently completed a 6-month phlebotomy-training program at a local vocational school. According to the hospital's own policies, her technique was to be observed for 40 hours before she could perform venipunctures unsupervised. After only two-and-a-half hours of supervised punctures, she was cleared to draw blood on her own. Two months later, she inflicted a permanent nerve injury on a patient during a venipuncture and the hospital was successfully sued for violations against the standard of care.
Commentary: Even with the best training and supervision protocol on the books, there is no effective defense for a facility that violates its own protocol when an injury results from a randomly implemented policy.

At the minimum, training programs must encompass instruction in the following areas:

➢Needle safety
➢Site selection
➢Anatomy of the antecubital
➢Equipment: syringe vs. tube holder
➢Mechanics of the venipuncture
➢Patient positioning
➢Site preparation
➢Maintaining support during the puncture
➢Correct angle of insertion
➢Exchanging tubes
➢Terminating the puncture
➢Recovering the failed puncture
➢The order in which tubes must be drawn
➢Labeling requirements
➢Secondary puncture sites
➢Patient considerations
➢Dietary considerations
➢Medication considerations
➢Capillary punctures
➢Minimum fill volumes
➢Specimen storage and transportation.

A phlebotomy-training program should consist of a written test and practical application of the skills learned. Both should evaluate the individual's knowledge of the critical elements of phlebotomy and at least assess the collector's knowledge pertaining to:

➢Site selection
➢Risks to the healthcare professional
➢Risks to the patient
➢Site preparation
➢Performing the puncture
➢Handling, storing, and transporting specimens.

An excellent text on establishing a phlebotomy-training program is *Phlebotomy Techniques: A Curriculum Guide* by Susan Phelan, MHS, MT(ASCP) (ASCP Press, 1998). For evaluating competency, *Phlebotomy/Blood Collection* by Kathleen Becan-McBride and Diana Garza (Appleton & Lange, 1998) includes sample test questions to guide healthcare professionals in drafting exams. (For information on obtaining these and other guides, see Appendix IV).

Adequate training and supervision is not enough, however. Complete documentation of those healthcare professionals who successfully complete the facility's phlebotomy training program must be maintained in order to demonstrate that phlebotomy skills are safely and effectively implemented. It's best to operate from the perspective of an inspector who assumes that "if it wasn't documented, it wasn't done."

> Annual evaluations of phlebotomy competency should be comprehensive and thorough. Both practical and written or oral examinations are necessary to assess skill and knowledge.

Establishing High Standards of Performance

In addition to completing a well-organized and well-implemented orientation program, those who perform phlebotomy should be evaluated regularly for technique. Bad habits inevitably creep in, especially if individuals do not perform punctures routinely. A well-established timetable of evaluation can prevent habits from developing that put patients at risk. "Regularly" can be whatever the facility defines it to be, but a written and practical evaluation 3 to 6 months after the person is cleared to perform unsupervised punctures and annually thereafter is sufficient. In fact, the annual evaluations can easily be incorporated into the employee's overall annual performance review. The same checklist used in their initial training can be used for evaluations in conjunction with a written and practical demonstration of the individual's phlebotomy knowledge and skill. Of course, even if trainers adhere to a well-rounded phlebotomy training and evaluation program, without documentation the efforts cannot be proven and the facility is exposed to significant liability.

Drafting Safe Phlebotomy Procedures

Minimizing the risk of accidental exposure and injury cannot be accomplished without practicing safe and approved phlebotomy technique. The National Committee for Clinical Laboratory Standards (NCCLS) establishes and maintains the standards of venipuncture performance and other laboratory procedures. Publication H3-A4, *Procedure for the Collection of Diagnostic Blood Specimens by Venipuncture* sets forth the standard by which all

Legislating Phlebotomy Certification

Several states have legislated minimum training requirements for those who perform phlebotomy. Recently, California enacted legislation mandating that those who perform phlebotomy must be certified as a phlebotomist or be certified in a profession that includes phlebotomy in its official "scope of practice," (i.e. nurses, physicians, clinical laboratory scientists, etc.) Certified nursing assistants are not exempt from the regulations and will need to be certified in phlebotomy to collect blood specimens unless they have experience in blood collection at the time the regulations become effective sometime in 2001. CNAs with experience will have three years to meet the certification requirements.

Louisiana has also has passed legislation requiring phlebotomy certification for individuals who draw blood in facilities that are not under the authority of a medical director licensed in that state.

venipunctures should be performed and provides detailed directions for collecting diagnostic specimens by venipuncture. Because this document is considered the industry standard, any deviations that put the patient and healthcare professional at risk will be difficult to defend in a court of law. Healthcare professionals drafting their own phlebotomy procedures would do well to rely heavily on this important standard. The document and its companion videotape are available from the NCCLS. (See Appendix IV).

In hospitals, however, the laboratory's existing phlebotomy procedure should already be in compliance with this national standard and can be adapted easily for inclusion in nursing manuals.

Implementing Protective Policies

In addition to incorporating protective practices detailed in the NCCLS standard H3-A4, healthcare facilities should make sure they implement policies and procedures that assure the safety of their employees and patients beyond the scope of this document. This includes compliance with OSHA's Bloodborne Pathogen Standard, which constitutes the federal government's regulations on exposure prevention, disposal of contaminated sharps, hazardous spill procedures, and the procedure for reporting and treating accidental needlesticks. Although not all facilities are subject to OSHA regulations, compliance helps ensure the safety of the healthcare professional. Deviations can have devastating effects on healthcare professionals

Policies and procedures must reflect applicable legislation and stress the OSHA Bloodborne Pathogen Standard to fully protect employees. Deviations can be costly to employees and employers.

who suffer the consequences of safety policies that exist on paper, but not in practice.

Engineering Controls

Even with proper attention paid to technique, standards, training, evaluation, and compliance with federal guidelines, accidents will happen, deviations will occur, and healthcare professionals will be accidentally punctured by contaminated sharps. Each accidental needlestick plunges the injured healthcare worker's life into chaos. Grief, shock, anxiety, panic, and sleepless nights all conspire to devastate the victim. The possibility of contracting hepatitis, HIV, or any of the 20-plus diseases that can be acquired from an accidental needlestick affects every aspect of the victim's personal, professional, and social life. Every accidental needlestick is a personal tragedy, a tragedy that can be prevented in many cases when facilities implement proper engineering controls.

Since exposure to bloodborne pathogens has become such a major risk to healthcare professionals, suppliers of blood collection devices have developed a multitude of innovative safety devices to protect those who use them from risk. Over 1000 patents have been issued in protective needle design, and many new devices are now available. (Some of these devices are discussed in Chapter 8.) Unfortunately, market forces during the 1990s prevented them from becoming widely available to healthcare professionals.[9] Irrationally high pricing, competitive manipulation of purchase agreements, industry politics, and an unwillingness for some administrators to make employee safety a priority have combined to keep these safety devices out of the hands of healthcare professionals. In 1999, however, the state of California became the first state to mandate the use of safety needles in healthcare facilities. Many other states and the U. S. Congress have since enacted similar legislation. (See box, "Needle Safety Legislation" on page 2.)

The National Campaign for Healthcare Worker Safety was established in 1996 by Lynda Arnold, a nurse who acquired HIV through an accidental needlestick while starting an IV. Since she began her campaign to convince healthcare facilities to pledge to protect their employees through the facility-wide use of safe needle devices, hundreds have made the commitment.

Converting a facility completely to safety needles for phlebotomy and IV therapy can cost a medium-size facility as little as $10,000;[10] for larger facilities the projection is $100,000 or more.[11] It has been shown that this expense can be offset by the resultant reduction in how much facilities pay to treat accidental needlesticks.[10] One

> Legislation and an increased awareness of the cost effectiveness of facility-wide use of safety needles are combining to reduce accidental needlesticks.

study reports that the cost of treating an employee infected with HIV while performing routine procedures can exceed $500,000.[12] The immediate cost to treat an accidental needlestick has been estimated to be up to $4000, including testing both patient and worker and administering HIV prophylaxis.[3] If the needlestick results in an acquired disease, the cost skyrockets. In the case of hepatitis, a liver transplant can cost an employer $150,000 or more; the average lawsuit for occupationally acquired HIV settles for $2 million to $5 million.[3] Armed with these estimates, managers and healthcare professionals can build a convincing case for administrators to purchase only needles that will offer their employees the most protective technology available for performing phlebotomy procedures.

A second important engineering control that can reduce a facility's accidental needlestick rate is the availability of a needle disposal unit at the point of use. The window of vulnerability to accidental needlesticks opens when the contaminated needle is removed from the patient's arm and closes when it is permanently concealed or discarded. Minimizing this window is essential to lowering a facility's frequency of accidental needlesticks. Therefore, healthcare professionals should have access to sharps containers at the point of use so that contaminated needles can be discarded immediately. Unfortunately, many facilities install sharps containers away from the point of use—for example, by the door in patients' rooms—thereby preventing immediate sharps disposal and facilitating accidental needlesticks. If a permanently installed sharps container is not within reach at the point of use, a portable unit should be included on the phlebotomy tray or otherwise carried to the patient's side.

> The window of vulnerability for sustaining an accidental needlestick opens when the contaminated needle is removed from the arm and does not close until it is discarded or permanently concealed.

In summary, when those new to phlebotomy take on this added responsibility, the safety of the healthcare professional and the patient can only be guaranteed by soliciting their input, establishing a comprehensive phlebotomy training protocol with high standards and regular performance evaluations, drafting procedures that incorporate sound and safe phlebotomy techniques, implementing policies that protect the healthcare professional from accidental needlesticks, and providing engineering controls that protect those performing phlebotomy procedures from injury.

It is the duty not only of the manager but the healthcare professional as well to make sure these criteria are met. By taking ownership in the process, a cooperative effort will most likely produce a successful outcome.

References

1 Jagger J. Risky procedure, risky devices, risky job. *Adv Exposure Prev.* 1994;1(1):4-9.

2 Carlsen W, Holding R. Epidemic ravages caregivers; thousands die from diseases contracted through needle sticks. *San Francisco Chronicle.* April 12, 1998.

3 Pallatroni L. Needlesticks: Who pays the price when costs are cut on safety? *MLO*, July 1998;30(7):30-35.

4 Kearsly S. High profits—at what cost? *San Francisco Chronicle.* http://sfgate.com. Accessed June 8, 1998.

5 Jagger J. Rates of needlestick injury caused by various devices in a university hospital. *N Engl J Med.*1988;319(5).

6 Holding, R, Carlsen, W. Watchdogs fail health workers. *San Francisco Chronicle.* http://sfgate.com. Accessed June 8, 1998.

7 International Healthcare Worker Safety Center. Risk of infection following a single HIV, HBV, or HCV-contaminated needlestick or sharp instrument injury. http://www.med.virginia.edu. Accessed August 2, 2000.

8 Perlman D, Takacs G. The 10 stages of change. *Nurs Manage.* April 1990;21(4)208-216.

9 Zweig P Zellner W. Locked out of the hospital. *Business Week.* March 16, 1998, pp 75-76.

10 Garvin M. Innovative new equipment lowers risks of needlesticks. *Health Facilities Manage.* 1996; 9(10).

11 Safer Needles Limit Injuries. *Healthcare Purchasing News.* March 1997.

12 Stock S. Universal precautions to prevent HIV transmission to healthcare workers: an economic analysis. *Can Med Assoc J.* 1990;142(9):932-946.

Chapter 2

Site Selection and Equipment

SITE SELECTION

Veins just under the anterior surface of the arm—opposite the elbow—are most commonly used to obtain blood. This area is known as the antecubital area. (*Ante* comes from the Latin word for "before"; *cubital* from the Latin for "elbow.") Because this site contains several large veins that are often close to the surface of the skin and, therefore, easily accessible, this site is the area of choice for venipunctures. However, many factors must be taken into consideration before selecting the antecubital area as the site for a venipuncture.

> Emotional and mental status of the patient—If restraint is necessary, veins in areas that are most easily immobilized offer the greater chance of obtaining specimens successfully. Because the antecubital area is in the joint of the arm, it may be difficult to immobilize. Thus, it may be prudent to draw from an alternative site.

> Prior mastectomies—If the patient has had a mastectomy, punctures in the arm on the same side are not permitted without physician approval. Significant lymph node removal often accompanies surgical mastectomy procedures. Because lymph nodes regulate fluid balance, their removal effectively interferes with lymph flow (lymphostasis) in the respective limb. Blood collected from the same side as a mastectomy will contain higher concentrations of lymphocytes and waste products normally contained in the lymph fluid.[1]

More importantly to the patient, any aggravation to the affected limb can result in excruciating pain from edema, which can last for months or years. Patients who have undergone mastectomies

The patient's emotional status and prior mastectomies must be taken into consideration when selecting the site for a venipuncture.

15

are also increasingly susceptible to infection in the affected limb from even the smallest breaks in the skin. Most mastectomy patients will be acutely aware of the potential complications and will inform the phlebotomist before a puncture is attempted. These circumstances should be taken seriously.

Case Study
A physician ordered an IV to be inserted on an inpatient who had undergone a prior mastectomy. She informed the nurse of the condition, but the nurse inserted the cannula into the affected arm nonetheless. The patient experienced a fluid imbalance in the limb resulting in excruciating pain and discomfort for months. She sued the facility that employed the nurse for violations against the standard of care.
Commentary: Punctures to the same side as a prior mastectomy should never be performed without the written permission of the patient's physician.

The availability of veins, collector's skill, and the presence of edema, injury, and IV infusion must also be considered in venipuncture site selection.

➢ Availability of veins—Anatomically speaking, most patients have six potentially acceptable veins in their combined antecubital areas. In some patients, though, it can be difficult to locate even one. Obesity can be a factor. However, occasionally nature's simple randomness produces an antecubital with veins that cannot be located. Although there is beauty in diversity, if you happen to be looking for a vein in such patients, there can also be frustration.

➢ Collector's skill—a lack of confidence in one's ability to puncture veins that are palpable, but not visible, moves many healthcare professionals new to phlebotomy to consider alternative sites. As one's phlebotomy skills improve, phlebotomists rely less on their sense of sight and more on their sense of touch to locate veins.

➢ Presence of edema—Venipunctures should be avoided in an arm with edema. Swelling makes locating veins more difficult and can prolong healing and closure of the puncture site. Excessive swelling can alter the composition of the blood passing through the affected limb.

➢ Injuries—Naturally, punctures in an arm that is injured, burned, scarred, or otherwise traumatized should be avoided. Likewise, infected or inflamed antecubital areas should not be considered. In geriatric patients, strokes may limit hyperextension of the arm, thereby preventing access to the antecubital area.

➢ Infusion of IV fluids—Contamination of specimens with IV fluids is one of the most common errors in specimen collection.

The literature is highly specific on the restrictions to phlebotomies performed on arms in which fluids are being infused. (See "Venipunctures and IV Infusions" on page 24).

If any of these conditions preclude the use of the antecubital area, an alternative site should be considered. (See Chapter 4.)

Surveying the Antecubital Area

Begin by tightening a tourniquet several inches above the bend in the arm. To assure patient comfort, the tourniquet should not roll into a rope-like constrictor, but remain flat against the skin around the circumference of the upper arm. It should be tight, though not uncomfortably so. A loop of the tourniquet should be tucked between the tourniquet and the arm so as to provide an easy, one-handed release (see Figures 2.1-2.6). A blood pressure cuff can be used in place of a tourniquet and inflated to 40 mm Hg.

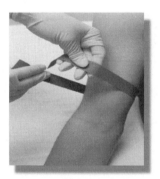

Figure. 2.1: Bring tourniquet around arm several inches above the intended puncture site.

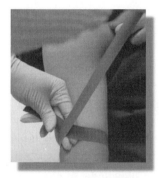

Figure. 2.2: Place two fingers under the end of the tourniquet held close to the patient.

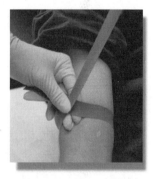

Figure. 2.3: Stretch the opposite end and hold with thumb until taut.

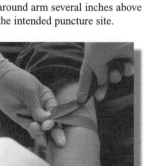

Figure. 2.4: Create an opening between tourniquet and skin by spreading the fingers apart.

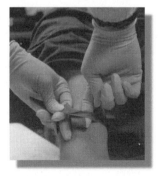

Figure. 2.5: Tuck a loop into opening from above.

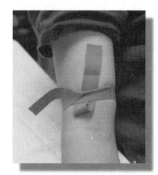

Figure. 2.6: Tourniquet should be snug and flat with the looped end out of the way and accessible for release.

Instruct the patient to make a fist, but discourage pumping of the fist as it can elevate levels of potassium and ionized calcium in the bloodstream.[2] It is also distracting and brings about movement in the antecubital area that interferes with locating the veins.

Identify the most prominent of the three acceptable veins in the area—the *median cubital*, *basilic* and *cephalic* (see Figure 2.7)—visually and by palpation. Although those new to phlebotomy may only feel confident puncturing veins that are visible, this is a luxury not all patients will present. Palpate for each vein by pushing lightly on the skin with increasing pressure using the index finger. Veins will feel spongy, resilient, and have a tube-like curvature. Tendons and bone will be hard and distinctively different. Attempt to locate the median cubital vein first.

> Of the three acceptable veins in the antecubital area for venipuncture, the median cubital vein is the vein of choice.

VEIN PALPATION: LIGHTLY PRESSING DOWN ON THE SKIN OF THE ANTECUBITAL AREA REPEATEDLY WITH VARYING DEGREES OF PRESSURE TO DETECT UNDERLYING VEINS. TOO MUCH PRESSURE MAY NOT ALLOW FOR THE TACTILE SENSATION OF THE VEIN'S CURVATURE OR ELASTICITY. LIKEWISE, TOO LITTLE PRESSURE MAY NOT BRING THE FINGER CLOSE ENOUGH TO FEEL THE VEIN.

Repeat palpation on the lateral (outer) aspect of the arm where the cephalic vein lies. Complete the survey by palpating the skin on the medial (inner) aspect of the antecubital area where the basilic vein lies. If veins are not obvious by sight or touch, repeat the survey on the opposite arm if it is accessible. You may not be able to locate all three veins; more than likely only one or two will be identifiable—perhaps none at all.

If it can be located, the vein of choice is the median cubital vein for several reasons:

1 Proximity—the median cubital vein is typically the closest to the skin's surface, making it readily accessible.
2 Immobility—the median cubital vein is also the most stationary of the three. This makes a successful puncture more probable.
3 Safety—punctures to the median cubital vein pose the least risk of injuring underlying structures.
4 Comfort—to the patient, the median cubital vein brings less discomfort when punctured. Although the vein itself has no innervation, the surface of the skin seems less sensitive there than it is over the cephalic and basilic veins.

☺First of four secrets to a painless venipuncture!

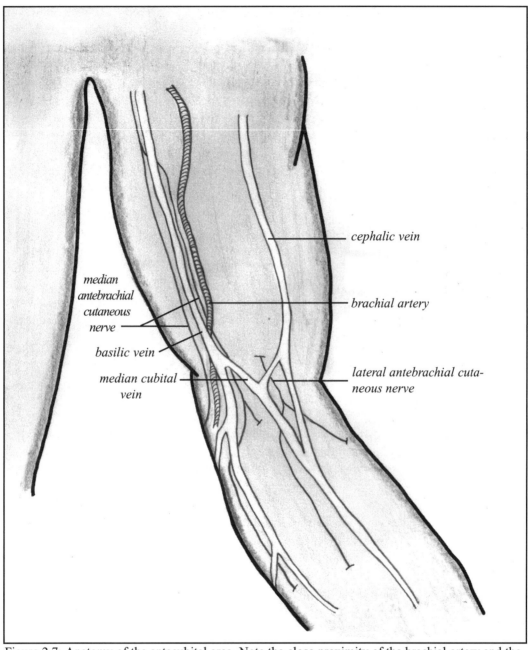

Figure 2.7: Anatomy of the antecubital area. Note the close proximity of the brachial artery and the branches of the medial antebrachial cutaneous nerve to the basilic vein. Punctures to this vein must carry a high degree of confidence that the vein will be accessed successfully and without probing.

The median cubital vein is only the vein of choice, however, if it is visible or palpable *and if there is a high degree of confidence that it can be accessed successfully.* Selecting an indistinct median cubital vein over one of the other clearly visible or palpable veins may result in an unsuccessful attempt and subject the patient to a second puncture. Likewise, choosing another vein over the median cubital when the median cubital is clearly present can put the patient at risk for injury.

Case Study

A phlebotomist was presented with the option of puncturing the median cubital vein or the basilic vein; both appeared to be accessible. She chose the basilic vein and, because of poor technique, subsequently pierced a nerve that resulted in permanent injury to the patient. Partly because the phlebotomist chose the basilic vein when the median cubital vein was a well-defined option—clearly identified in most texts as the vein of choice—the jury found the phlebotomist in error and awarded nearly $50,000 to the patient.

Commentary: It is acceptable to puncture any of the three veins in the antecubital area. But if the collector has poor technique or resorts to probing, the basilic vein is the least forgiving.

Collectors who select a vein in the antecubital area other than the median cubital vein should be aware of the risks involved and be prepared to defend their selection should poor technique result in an injury.

Even though collectors should select the vein that offers the highest degree of confidence, those who choose a vein other than the median cubital should be aware of the risks involved. In the absence of a prominent median cubital vein, the cephalic vein should be considered next. Drawing blood from the basilic vein brings the greatest risk to the patient because of underlying structures. Branches of the median cubital antebrachial cutaneous nerve can nestle against this vein. Once pierced, these nerves send shooting pain down the length of the limb to the fingers and up to the shoulder and chest. If the injury is severe, nerve injury can be permanent. Most nerve injuries that result from punctures in the antecubital area are from errant attempts to puncture the basilic vein

In addition to nerves, the basilic vein's close proximity to the brachial artery subjects the patient to the risk of an arterial nick and subsequent hemorrhage. Should the healthcare professional involve this artery unknowingly, the consequences to the patient can range from a barely perceptible bruising to severe hemorrhaging. If undetected, hemorrhaging can be so severe that it results in a compression nerve injury from the interstitial pressure or necessitates amputation of the limb. Therefore, when considering punctures to the inside aspect of the antecubital area, collectors should attempt to locate the brachial artery by feeling for a pulse and avoid punctures in the area if the artery lies precariously close to the basilic vein.

Case Study
A nurse at a blood donor station attempted to obtain a unit of blood from a basilic vein that was palpable, but not visible. She was initially unsuccessful and attempted to manipulate the 16 gauge needle into the vein. The attempt was unsuccessful, and the donor was sent home. Later in the day, the individual's arm swelled and became so painful that he went to the emergency room. The ER physician diagnosed a compression injury to the nerves secondary to an arterial nick that hemorrhaged into his arm. The lingering nerve injury brought a lawsuit against the facility.
Commentary: Injuries don't just happen with 16 gauge needles. All punctures should be performed with careful consideration for underlying structures.

Regardless of the size of the needle, the risk of injury while accessing the basilic vein is *moderate* whenever the vein is not visible and *high* when it is neither visible nor palpable. A moderate risk, however, shouldn't preclude the use of this vein for the collection of blood specimens; often the basilic is the patient's most prominent vein. Healthcare professionals must be aware, however, of the risk in accessing this vein and use it only when no other vein in the antecubital area is more accessible.

Case Study
A nurse was attempting to collect a unit of blood from the basilic vein with a 16 gauge needle. When there was no initial blood flow, she began probing the area, eventually piercing the median nerve and causing permanent damage, which brought a lawsuit against the blood donation facility.
Commentary: Punctures to the basilic vein should only be performed when there is a high degree of confidence that the vein will be accessed successfully. Side-to-side probing to relocate a missed vein should never be attempted.

In The Lab ➤━━━━━━━━➤ Diluted Specimen = Diluted Results

Specimens that come into the laboratory diluted with IV fluids aren't always obvious to the tech performing the test. In fact, only the most grossly diluted specimens will arouse suspicion. For some tests, like potassium or hemoglobin, grossly diluted specimens can elevate or depress laboratory values to levels inconsistent with life. Conversely, diluted specimens to be tested for therapeutic drugs, toxicology screens, and the like can produce negative or normal results when the patient's actual level is positive or dangerously elevated.

For example, Let's say Mr. Smith, a new patient, has his blood drawn for a metabolic profile, toxicology screen, hepatitis profile, and CBC. The collector draws the blood above an active IV site unaware that it is unacceptable to do so (see "Drawing Above an IV" on page 24). When the specimen is sent to the laboratory for processing and distribution, processors immediately send the CBC tube to hematology and set the red top aside for clotting to complete (10 to 30 minutes). Once clotted, it is centrifuged for 5 to 10 minutes to separate the serum for the remaining tests.

The serum is removed and divided into three separate transfer tubes: one to the chemistry department for the metabolic profile, another to the toxicology lab for the toxicology screen, and the third to special chemistry for the hepatitis profile. Before the serum arrives in any of the other departments, the hematology department, having already tested the specimen, calls the physician with a hemoglobin of 5.9, which it had confirmed by repeat testing. The physician responds by adding a type and crossmatch to the orders.

While the toxicology lab and special chemistry department test their respective aliquots of serum, the tech in the chemistry department has completed the metabolic profile and is now reviewing the results. The potassium level reads at 7.9—a level incompatible with life—and must be confirmed by repeat testing. Meanwhile, the toxicology lab has finished its testing and is reporting negative results on all metabolites. Mr. Smith is having his blood drawn again, this time for the type and crossmatch, a process that requires a special patient identification protocol that was not in place during the first draw. ➤━━➤

Repeat testing of the potassium confirms the elevated level. The chemistry tech notices that the glucose, sodium, and chloride levels are also significantly elevated. However, all other levels are well below normal or at the low end of the normal range. Because of the erratic results, the tech calls the floor and discusses the results with the nurse. Together they make the connection between the elevated analytes obtained by the analyzer and the fluids being infused— D_5W, KCl, and normal saline. The collector is questioned on the draw site, and it is discovered that the specimen was drawn above the IV and, therefore, diluted by fluids.

It has been over an hour since the initial order was placed, and the physician has called the lab three times for the rest of the results. Mr. Smith is failing fast. The chemistry tech investigates other tests ordered at the same time and alerts the hematology department, toxicology lab, and special chemistry section that the prior specimen was diluted and the results should be invalidated. The hematologist and toxicologist collaborate and notify the physician of the erroneous results. After bellowing in fits consistent with bovine labor, the physician puts the type and crossmatch on hold and orders a flurry of incident reports filled out. Mr. Smith's blood is collected a third time.

After processing, centrifugation, and distribution, the results from the fresh specimen eventually show normal hemoglobin, potassium, glucose, sodium, and chloride levels. All liver enzymes—previously at the low end of normal because of the dilution—are elevated. The toxicology screen is positive for alcohol and barbiturates and the hepatitis panel is positive for hepatitis B; initially, all were negative from the dilution factor.

As you can see from this scenario, poor judgment in a specimen collection site initiated a cascade of actions, reactions, and delays that could have been prevented. Two additional collections, which would have been otherwise unnecessary, confirmatory testing, repeat testing, delays in treatment, and a blizzard of paperwork all translate into an expensive waste of supplies, equipment and human resources. And that's not to mention the incalculable cost to Mr. Smith from the delay in treatment and diagnosis. Adding further to the total cost was the strain the incident placed on the relationships among the physician, the nursing department, and the laboratory.

In summary, select the median cubital vein when presented with two veins that appear equally accessible. Consider the basilic vein only when punctures to either the median cubital or the cephalic vein on either arm are less likely to be successful.

Venipunctures and IV Infusions

Drawing above an IV site

Draws from above an active IV should never be performed, even if the flow of IV fluids is momentarily interrupted.

Fluids infusing in the hand, wrist, or forearm can corrupt any blood specimen collected in the antecubital area of that arm. The result is a diluted blood specimen that contains fluids, medications, electrolytes, donor blood, glucose, and/or any number of compounds and can yield laboratory results completely inconsistent with the patient's actual metabolic state. Some collectors feel that temporarily interrupting an active IV prior to a draw above the infusion site is acceptable. However, one study showed that shutting off an IV for 3 minutes and drawing above the infusion-site will falsely elevate results if the analytes tested also existed in the IV fluid that had been entering the vein.[10] Therefore, *it is against the standards of phlebotomy to perform a venipuncture above an active IV site,* even if it has been recently discontinued. In fact, NCCLS recommends that venipunctures be avoided from previously active infusion sites for 24 to 48 hours after the infusion was discontinued to eliminate potential sources of test error. Never attempt to trace the vein in which fluids are being infused with the intent to collect blood from another vein. The circuitous nature of the circulatory system makes such presumptions impossible.

Case Study

The lab at a midsize hospital called a nurse with a panic level PTT on one of her patients. She discontinued the patient's heparin therapy for 1 hour, then followed protocol by restarting it at a slower rate. After 6 hours, a repeat PTT was drawn and the results showed subtherapeutic levels. Questioning the validity of the earlier result, she asked the patient where the phlebotomist drew the first specimen. He pointed to a recent puncture mark just above the IV.

Commentary: This is a case in which the patient's anticoagulant therapy was unnecessarily interrupted, making him vulnerable to stroke or other complications of blood clot formation because of a specimen collection error.

Case Study

A physician ordered stat blood work on a woman who went into seizures 2 days after surgery. The results were so extreme that the physician accused the phlebotomist of drawing blood above the IV site. Within hours, the patient coded and expired. The physician named in the wrongful death suit blamed the phlebotomist, claiming that if the specimen was drawn properly, the results would have enabled him to save the patient. The lab results from the draw did not support the accusation, and the phlebotomist was exonerated.

Commentary: Although it was proven that the phlebotomist could not have drawn the blood from above the IV site, this case illustrates the types of accusations collectors may have to defend themselves against. Knowing and applying the basic principles of blood collection are critical to defend against such frivolous charges.

Drawing below an IV site

The consensus in the literature leans toward avoiding draws below an active IV unless absolutely necessary. However, it is conceivable that circumstances can preclude venous access in any other site. In the absence of other acceptable sites, a venipuncture below an active IV can be performed minimizing specimen contamination if the following steps are taken:[2-10]

> Draws below an active IV should only be performed as a last resort and done so with adherence to a very specific procedure.

1) Shut off the IV for 2 minutes prior to the puncture
2) Tighten the tourniquet below the IV site and above the intended puncture site
3) Perform the puncture as usual, but discard the first 5 cc of blood
4) Document that the puncture was performed below an active IV site.

SUPPLIES AND EQUIPMENT

In preparing for a venipuncture, it is important to assemble the materials and gather the supplies so that they are within easy reach during the procedure. Using a fully stocked phlebotomy tray keeps supplies organized and at hand. The tray of supplies and equipment should include all materials necessary to perform the procedure with supplies necessary react to potential complications.

Supplies should at least include:

- 2x2 inch gauze or cotton balls
- 70 % isopropyl alcohol preps
- 22 or 23 gauge needles for syringes
- 22 or 23 gauge needles for tube holders
- A variety of syringe sizes
- Tube holder for vacuum-assisted draws
- Winged-infusion (butterfly) sets

- Tourniquets
- Bandages
- Gloves
- Sharps container
- An assortment of collection tubes
- Marking pen

> Collectors concerned with the patient's comfort should collect specimens with a needle no larger than a 22 gauge.

It is important, however, not to place supplies on the patient's bed where they are likely to be swept off by sudden movements. Also avoid placing phlebotomy trays on the patient's bedside tray. From a standpoint of infection control, the bottom of the phlebotomy tray likely contains a host of pathogenic microorganisms. If the tray is placed on the same table that the patient eats from, leans on, and holds his/her personal belongings (eyeglasses, hearing aids, dentures, etc) it brings that patient in direct contact with a multitude of potentially infectious bacteria. Instead, put the tray on a chair or other elevated stand that can be pulled within reach.

Needle Selection

Although some needles are useful only in a limited capacity, a broad variety of sizes exists for venipuncture use. The largest of these needles, 16 to 19 gauge, are reserved for drawing large quantities of blood, for example, blood donor units or in therapeutic phlebotomy in which an entire unit of blood is drawn from a patient. Although readily available, 20 gauge needles are too large and painful for routine phlebotomy.

☺Second of four secrets to a painless venipuncture!

The most common needle used is the 21 gauge needle. Its bore is still relatively large, however, and those concerned with the patient's comfort should avoid using this needle size in favor of the 22 gauge needle. This size is ideal for most punctures because it provides a good blood flow with little or no discomfort to the patient upon insertion when the proper technique is used. The 23 gauge needle is an excellent choice for pediatric draws, hand veins, or veins that appear fragile or problematic. It is ideal for children because its size provides an extra measure of comfort. Because of its small bore, the needle is less likely to collapse the small, delicate hand veins of adults or to collapse or traumatize the fragile veins of geriatric patients.

Collectors should avoid the use of 25 gauge needles as the small bore may result in the *hemolysis* of the red blood cells (RBCs) as they pass through, especially if a vacuum or excessive syringe pressure is applied.

HEMOLYSIS—THE RUPTURE OF RBCS DURING COLLECTION,
HANDLING, STORAGE, OR TRANSPORTATION, RESULTING IN CON-
TAMINATION AND TINGEING OF THE SERUM OR PLASMA WITH
THE HEMOGLOBIN PIGMENT. (SEE "IN THE LAB" BOX, PAGE 29.)

Tube Holders, Syringes, and Winged-Infusion Sets

One of the first decisions blood collectors have to make is whether to use a tube holder for vacuum-assisted draws, a syringe, or a winged-infusion ("butterfly") set to collect the specimen. Often the site selected for the puncture will dictate the equipment to be used. Each system has its benefits and drawbacks, including safety, cost, and ease-of-use.

Tube holders

If the vein selected is prominent and in the antecubital area, a vacuum-assisted draw using a tube holder is the most convenient and cost-effective method. With vacuum-assisted draws, once the needle is in place, tubes are quickly and effortlessly filled. This system offers both convenience and ease of use, which appeal to many healthcare professionals. Originally intended to be reusable, conventional tube holders are inexpensive to use and reduce the quantities of supplies that must be brought to the patient. However, increasing concerns over safety and tube holder contamination are making their reuse an issue (see box "Re-Using Tube Holders" on page 28 and "OSHA's Stance on Needle Recapping and Removal" on page 137).

Additionally, vacuum assisted draws are not appropriate for use on all veins on all patients. Although the benefits of tube holders are undisputed on prominent veins in the antecubital area (where most venipunctures take place), they have limited usefulness on smaller veins in other areas.

Unlike syringe draws, the use of tube holders does not allow collectors to control the vacuum pressure applied to the inside of the vein. After needle insertion, the vacuum that exists in the tube pulls the specimen from the vein into the tube. Once the tube is applied, the full force of the vacuum within the tube is transferred to the interior of the vein. Even though the vacuum decreases proportionally as the

> Tube holders should only be used when drawing blood from the antecubital area.

Re-Using Tube Holders

Studies have shown that tube holders become contaminated with trace amounts of blood even after one use.[11,12] OSHA states in its Bloodborne Pathogen Standard (BPS) that removing needles from collection devices after use (and, therefore, reusing tube holders) is not allowed unless no alternative is feasible or is required by the specific medical procedure. In such cases the needle must be recapped through the use of a mechanical device or a one-handed technique.[13] Because of the contamination issue and the BPS, facilities should consider discarding or cleansing tube holders after one use with a 10 % bleach solution. Healthcare professionals are advised to follow their facility's policy regarding the re-use of tube holders. (See "OSHA's Stance on Recapping and Removing Needles on page 137.)

---

tube fills, the initial application of the vacuum to the inside of the vein can be enough to collapse the vein when there is not enough space between the beveled opening of the needle and the inner wall of the vein. This often occurs in small veins or when the needle is not fully within the vein. Instead of pulling blood through the needle, the vacuum pulls the wall of the vein itself on to the beveled opening, occluding it and preventing blood from passing through the needle into the tube. Sometimes, changing to a smaller tube, which contains less vacuum, can salvage the venipuncture. However, it's best to understand the limitations of the equipment when selecting the puncture site. Therefore, because pressure is harder to control while using tube holders, they should only be used on the large-diameter veins of the antecubital area or on smaller veins only when smaller tubes are available.

> Tube holders do not allow users to control the force of the draw and can result in collapsed veins.

Syringes

The most important benefit of using a syringe is that it affords the operator the ability to control the pressure being applied inside the vein. This control is essential in veins of small diameter and veins that appear fragile or otherwise difficult to access. Because the beveled opening of the needle may be in close proximity to the inside wall of the vein—a condition that causes the collapse of the vein when using a vacuum-assisted system—the collector can pull back on the plunger as slowly as necessary to maintain blood flow into the barrel of the syringe. Should the pressure of pulling the plunger become excessive during the collection and collapse the vein, the operator has the ability to reduce the pulling pressure, which can release the occlusion and restore blood flow into the syringe. This

The Evils of Hemolysis ◄─────────────────◄ In the Lab

When a specimen becomes hemolyzed during the collection process, it becomes evident only when the specimen is centrifuged and the serum is separated from the cellular components of blood. However, if the specimen collected is for a test for which separation is not necessary (eg, CBCs), hemolysis can go undetected and its effect on the results may never be known. For example, specimens collected for CBCs are not centrifuged since the sample to be tested must remain well-mixed. Because hemolysis is the rupturing of RBCs, gross hemolysis results in an RBC count that is falsely decreased for two reasons: 1) the physical destruction of cells and 2) the dilution effect that occurs when the liquid content of the RBCs (hemoglobin) is released.

For testing in which centrifugation is necessary (eg, red top tubes), hemolysis becomes evident by the red tinge it imparts to the serum. Not all hemolyzed specimens need to be re-collected, however, the necessity for which depends upon the test(s) that will be performed on the tinged serum. Testing in which hemolysis falsely elevates results include: potassium, LDH, AST, ALT, phosphorous, magnesium and ammonia. Values that are falsely lowered by hemolysis include RBC counts, hemoglobin, and hematocrit.[2,15] For many tests, however, the interference of hemolysis is a function of the test methodology the testing facility is using to perform the assay. For example, one laboratory may employ a method of obtaining protime results for which hemolysis interferes, while another laboratory may employ a method immune from the interfering factor of free hemoglobin. For this reason, one should rely on the specimen rejection criteria established by the testing facility.

For specimens tested in facilities remote to the site of collection (ie, long-term care facilities, physicians' offices without labs, etc), healthcare professionals may not learn of the necessity for re-collection for a day or more. Often this creates hardships and impossibilities that cannot be overcome, underscoring the importance of utilizing good technique while collecting specimens to minimize the potential for this scenario.

ability to control the pressure is critical to successful punctures on smaller diameter veins and on veins outside the antecubital area.

However, if the needle is not completely in the vein and blood fills the barrel of the syringe too slowly, excessive pulling pressure on the plunger can hemolyze RBCs rendering the specimen unacceptable. In addition, a specimen that is collected too slowly can begin to clot in the barrel of the syringe. This condition cannot only make it difficult to evacuate the specimen into the collection tubes when the puncture is complete, but can also introduce micro-clots into the specimen and lead to erroneous results. If needle placement is inaccurate, an attempt to readjust the needle to accommodate a better flow is preferred over a slow, high-pressure draw. (See "Recovering the Failed Venipuncture," on page 56.)

A final benefit not afforded with the vacuum-assisted system is the visible "flash" of blood into the hub of the syringe that often occurs when the vein has been accessed. Many healthcare professionals rely on this flash exclusively as an indication of a successful puncture. However, the absence of a flash of blood into the hub does not necessarily indicate the needle is not in place. Low blood pressure, a loose tourniquet, and other factors prevent this from being a completely reliable indicator of vein penetration. Therefore, nursing personnel should be careful in using this as exclusive proof of vein accession.

There are serious disadvantages to using syringes that all healthcare professionals should consider when selecting equipment. Syringes used in conjunction with standard needles without safety features are associated with a high rate of accidental needlesticks. In many settings, concealment of the needle and disposal of the assembly are often difficult to accomplish immediately. Therefore, syringe and standard needle combinations should not be used where a vacuum-assisted collection is possible.

Winged-infusion "butterfly" sets

Winged-infusion sets, also known as "butterfly" sets, find favor with many healthcare professionals as blood collection devices; many use them exclusively. The greatest benefit is their lightweight design, which makes them easy to manipulate. In addition, the wings allow for a lower angle and greater control of insertion than what a syringe or tube holder can allow. Like syringes, winged-infusion sets allow the operator to see an immediate "flash" of blood in the tubing, indicating that the vein has been successfully accessed. This feature, as with syringes, offers an assurance that using a vacuum-assisted

> Syringes allow collectors to see the flash of blood upon venous access, indicating the needle is in place. However, syringe use is associated with a higher risk of accidental needlestick rate than the use of tube holders.

device does not. As mentioned earlier, though, the absence of this flash does not mean that the needle is improperly positioned within the vein.

However convenient, butterfly sets have significant drawbacks to their use as routine devices for blood collection. The healthcare professional concerned with minimizing the discomfort of a venipuncture need only compare the bevel of the winged-infusion set with the bevel of the standard needle. The cut of a butterfly needle is much more blunt than that of standard needles and can result in a more painful puncture. Other drawbacks in using butterfly sets are that they are considerably more expensive to use than conventional devices, are too short to reach deep veins, and are associated with an inordinately high rate of accidental needlesticks. This last drawback is of great concern. Because the butterfly device has such a long tubing, it must be awkwardly dangled over, and carefully lowered into, a sharps container for disposal. This awkwardness puts the healthcare professional at increased risk for an accidental needlestick. One study showed that winged-infusion sets were responsible for 35% of all accidental needlesticks to phlebotomists.[14] Although some butterfly sets are available with a safety shield designed to protect the healthcare worker, for many who use the device, this shield takes two hands to activate, therefore limiting its effectiveness. Healthcare professionals should avoid using these devices unless special circumstances make them necessary.

> Of all phlebotomy equipment, butterfly sets are associated with the highest risk of accidental needlestick. Collectors who use them frequently should consider becoming proficient with the use of syringes and tube holders for their own safety.

EQUIPMENT ASSEMBLY

Tube Holders

Needles for vacuum-assisted draws have a paper seal to assure their sterility. Before use, inspect the seal. If broken, discard the needle and select one in which the seal is intact. Hold opposite ends of the sealed needle with both hands and twist the two sections apart. Discard the shorter of the two plastic sheaths, leaving the needle itself still encased. Thread the exposed end, a short needle encased in a tight-fitting vinyl sleeve, into the open end of the threaded tube holder. If at any point in the assembly of any needle system, the needle is exposed and comes in contact with any surface, its sterility is lost and the needle must be discarded.

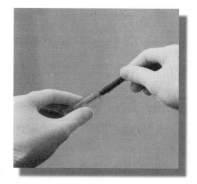

Figure 2.8: Assembling needle and tube holder.

Syringes

If choosing a syringe for the venipuncture, make sure the sterility of the syringe has not been compromised. This can be done in two ways:

1) Inspect the outer wrapper to assure it has not been opened. If the syringe is packaged in a protective hard-plastic casing, be certain the seal is intact by listening for an audible *click* when twisting to remove.

2) Make sure the plunger seal is not broken. Plungers on unused syringes should be seated and offer some resistance when used for the first time. Push or pull on the plunger to unseat. If there is initial resistance, followed by a freeing from the seal, the sterility of the device is assured providing the packaging is intact as above. If the resistance cannot be detected, discard the syringe and test another.

Select the appropriate needle size (see "Needle Selection" on page 26), and remove it from its packaging. If the packaging is not intact, the sterility of the needle cannot be guaranteed and the needle should be discarded. Assemble the needle onto the syringe, leaving the protective sheath in place until ready to perform the puncture.

> Winged infusion sets should always be used in conjunction with a tube holder when collecting directly into collection tubes.

Winged-Infusion Sets

Butterfly sets should always be used in conjunction with a syringe or tube holder. Inspect the package of the butterfly set. If previously opened, discard it and use an unopened set. To attach a syringe to a butterfly set, unseat the plunger of the syringe and advance it fully forward, expelling the air from the barrel of the syringe. Then simply attach the luer end of the butterfly set to the tip of the syringe. (Some sets come with adapters for vacuum-assisted draws, which must be removed from the luer before installing the syringe.)

To use a winged-infusion set for a vacuum-assisted draw, thread the adapter (usually attached to the luer end of the set) into the tube holder.

References

1 Phelan S. Q&A. *Lab Med.* 1999; 30(2): 93.

2 Dale J. Preanalytic variables in laboratory testing. *Lab Med.*1998;29(9):540-545.

3 Watson R, O'Kell R, Joyce J. Data regarding blood drawing sites in patients receiving intravenous fluids. *Am J Clin Pathol.* 1983;79(1):119-121.

4 Pendergraph G, Pendergraph C. *Handbook of Phlebotomy and Patient Service Techniques.* Baltimore, MD: Williams & Wilkins;1998.

5 Hoeltke L. *Phlebotomy: The Clinical Laboratory Manual Series.*Albany, NY: Delmar; 1995.

6 Hoeltke L. *The Complete Textbook of Phlebotomy.* Albany, NY:Delmar; 1994.

7 Kovanda B. *Multiskilling: Phlebotomy Collection Procedures for the Health Care Provider.* Albany, NY: Delmar; 1998.

8 Garza D, Becan-McBride K. *Phlebotomy Handbook.* 5th Ed. Stamford, CT: Appleton & Lange; 1999.

9 National Committee for Clinical Laboratory Standards (NCCLS). *Procedures for the Collection of Diagnostic Blood Specimens by Venipuncture.* Approved Standard, H3-A4, Villanova, PA:NCCLS; June, 1998.

10 Read D, Huberto V, Arkin C. Effect of drawing blood specimens proximal to an in-place but discontinued intravenous solution. *Am J Clin Pathol.* 1988;90(6):702-706.

11 Howanitz P, Schifman R. Phlebotomists' safety practices. *Arch Pathol Lab Med.* 1994;18:957-962.

12 Weinstein S, Hamrahi V, Popat A. et al. Blood contamination of reusable needle holders. *Am J Infect Control.* 1991;19(2).

13 US Department of Labor and Occupational Safety and Health Administration (OSHA). Occupational exposure to bloodborne pathogens; final rule (29 CFR 1910.1030). *Federal Register.*1991;Dec 6:64004-64182.

14 Jagger J. Risky procedure, risky devices, risky job. *Adv Exposure Prev* 1994; 1(1):4-9.

15 Becan-McBride K. Preanalytical phase an important requisite of laboratory testing. *Adv Med Lab Professionals.* Sept. 28, 1998:12-17.

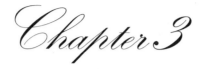

Chapter 3

The Venipuncture

Test Orders

In most states, all blood tests must be ordered and signed by a physician. Inspectors from certifying and accrediting agencies look for compliance with this standard. If the physician places a verbal order for the test, it must be documented as such on the patient's chart and later signed by the ordering physician. However, in emergencies where the patient's life is in danger, there is not always time to secure the physician's permission to order lab tests. Whenever nurses order tests in anticipation of the physician's approval, the order must be written in the patient's chart and eventually approved by the physician through a signature. Accreditation and certifying agencies can cite facilities that chart and charge for tests without signed orders.

> All blood tests must be ordered by physicians except in states where patients also have the right to order their own blood work.

Bedside Etiquette

It is important to approach phlebotomy from the perspective of the patient. Nursing personnel who are sensitive to patients' emotions are successful in making the phlebotomy experience a simple, forgettable procedure. Those who are insensitive stand the chance of upsetting patients, failing to obtain specimens, and provoking patients to be so irascible that they refuse the draw altogether.

Most healthcare professionals know that people have apprehensions about invasive procedures, even those as simple as a venipuncture. For many patients, allaying the fear of phlebotomy can be difficult. Because patient apprehension is impossible to predict, it is best that nursing personnel approach each patient as if the procedure brings great anxiety.

Patients in hospitals require the most compassion. Often they are ushered into unfamiliar surroundings, stripped of their personal effects, and find themselves without privacy, dignity, or power over what happens to them. They are inspected, examined, prodded, probed, and questioned on the most intimate details of their personal lives. They are given embarrassing garments to wear and denied most of the freedoms they took for granted in the outside world—sometimes even the freedom to get out of bed without permission. A multitude of strange faces comes and goes, each with a mandated interest in their bodies or bodily functions that, if pursued anywhere outside of a hospital, would be considered insulting and an invasion of privacy. Healthcare professionals who are aware of this perceived "institutionalizing" of the patient can be viewed as a refreshing exception to the patient's hospital experience.

Demonstrating respect for the privacy and dignity all patients deserve during hospitalization invites patients to be cooperative.

Begin by knocking on the patient's door. This shows that you respect the few square feet to which the patient has been confined. If the curtain is pulled, ask permission to enter so as not to embarrass the patient who may be using a bedpan, urinal, or bedside commode. If this is the case and the blood draw is not urgent, give the patient some time by offering to come back later. For nurses, clinical nursing assistants (CNAs), or other healthcare professionals who interact with the patient many times in the course of the day, knocking upon every single entry into a patient's room may be awkwardly repetitive and unnecessary. These professionals should take advantage of other

---

Preparing the Patient

The fear of the unknown, especially in children, can be paralyzing. (See Chapter 5, "Capillary Punctures, Pediatric Venipunctures.") Explaining the procedure to apprehensive patients can put them at ease. However, the terminology you use is critical. When preparing the patient for the puncture, avoid such inflammatory phrasing as "This is going to sting" or "hurt." Instead, warn of the impending puncture by using more subtle, yet equally accurate terms such as "You're going to feel a little poke." Use the words "pinch," "stick," or "mosquito bite" to equate the sensation to something familiar, but not intimidating.

While demonstrating the procedure on apprehensive patients, it may help to simulate the sensation they will feel by pinching the skin at the intended puncture site as an accurate predictor of the sensation. *By no means, however, should patients be told they won't feel anything!* Although it is possible to perform a painless venipuncture, if it turns out to be painful, a false representation can foster a lack of trust, complicating the next venipuncture on the same patient.

opportunities to show respect for the patient's privacy and dignity. Such courtesies restore an element of dignity to patients and contribute to their overall experience during hospitalization. Healthcare personnel who show respect for patients in this way will find them to be more cooperative for venipunctures and less likely to be frustrated should second attempts to obtain blood become necessary.

Regardless of the setting, those who are new to the patient should begin with identifying themselves and their purpose. Those who have already established a rapport with the patient need only identify their purpose. An attempt should be made to arouse patients who appear asleep or sedated.

If the patient expresses an interest in knowing the nature of the tests that are to be performed on the blood specimens drawn, healthcare professionals should attempt explanations in layperson's terms. If the patient presses for further information or if the collector is unsure of the nature of the test(s), suggest that the patient refer to the nurse or ordering physician for clarification.

If the patient verbalizes or demonstrates an apprehension about the procedure, it may be prudent to explain the steps of the procedure before performing the puncture. Once the procedure begins, distracting attention from the procedure with casual conversation can serve to calm the patient.

> Because arm bracelets can have erroneous information, collectors should verify identification more than one way to ensure the intended patient is being drawn.

Patient Identification

Few errors are more indefensible than misidentifying a patient. Treating a patient based on another's lab work can have devastating effects on patient management and bring a tempest of legal proceedings against the facility.

Inpatient identification.

The healthcare professional must ensure that the specimen drawn will be from the intended patient. Relying on arm bracelets alone is not sufficient. One study showed that up to 16 percent of arm bracelets have erroneous information.[1] The proper form of patient identification for inpatient venipunctures is to ask the patient to state his/her name, address, identification number, and/or birth date and compare it with the information on the order requisition and arm bracelet.[2] If the patient is unconscious or unable to respond, ask a member of the patient's care team or family to verify the patient's identification and compare it with the order requisition and arm bracelet. Document the name of the verifier.

If the arm bracelet is not attached to the patient, it is invalid and cannot be used. Even if the identifying bracelet is attached to the bed, it does not constitute reliable identification of the individual in the bed. Identification bracelets attached to the bedrail identify the bedrail, not the patient. Likewise, names written on water pitchers, bed tags, or posted charts do not constitute valid patient identification.

In confirming patients' names by soliciting a verbal response, the collector must ask patients to state their name in full. This must come in the form of the question: "Could you tell me your name, please?" Asking patients to affirm their name as in "Are you John Smith?" is not acceptable. Any patient in any state of consciousness can respond in the affirmative.

Under no circumstances should the patient's identity be assumed on the basis of his/her location. For example, a document containing a test order shows the patient, "John Williams," to be in "Bed 3." If the patient in Bed 3 is incoherent or unresponsive and does not have an identifying bracelet affixed to his/her person, it is dangerous to assume that John Williams is indeed the patient lying in Bed 3. In this case, it is the collector's duty to find someone responsible for the patient and verify the patient's identity. The verifier's name must be documented in the event that the patient is misidentified.

> All patients must be identified by a permanent or temporary identifier attached to their body in the form of an arm or ankle bracelet. Bracelets attached to bed rails or detached from the patient are invalid forms of identification.

The risk of patient misidentification is highest in hospital emergency departments (ED) where a flurry of activity descends upon traumatized patients. Here, blood collection can occur before hard patient identification is in place in the form of an arm bracelet or identifying tag. Although it may be pragmatic to rely on verbal identification from the ED team until such devices can be applied, it is best that a temporary number or other identifier is assigned and affixed around the patient's wrist or ankle until more exact information can be obtained. Policies that seek to affix temporary identifiers immediately to every patient upon entry to the ED can dramatically reduce patient identification errors. As with inpatient identification, patients unable to speak their names and without reliable identification must be identified by a healthcare professional responsible for the patient.

The information contained on a patient's arm bracelet should be compared to the hard copy of the order for the blood test that identifies the patient and what tests are to be drawn. This hard copy can come in the form of preprinted labels, a work list, or another form that puts down in writing the name of the patient, the location of the patient, the date and time of intended collection, and the tests that are to be collected. Any discrepancies must be investigated and resolved before the specimen is collected. In addition to comparing the patient's name, a second identifier should be used to match the order with the intended patient to protect against cases in which two patients have the same name. Supplemental identification in the form of a hospital number, medical records number, and the like can be used for this purpose.

Outpatient identification.
Healthcare professionals should not rely completely on the papers that an outpatient brings to the drawing station for identification. Outpatients should be asked to state their name in full, and their response should be compared with the orders and/or forms they have brought with them. Outpatients being collected for possible transfusions should be identified with an arm bracelet containing unique identifiers that establish and maintain their identification for possible transfusion at a later time.

Positioning Supplies and Equipment
Healthcare personnel should have a collection of venipuncture supplies and equipment within reach when drawing blood specimens. If more guaze or tubes are needed during the puncture, reaching for supplies that are not within arm's length puts the patient at risk of injury. Likewise, dropped supplies or equiment should not be used on a patient even if sterility has not been compromised. The perception to the patient is that the collector used contaminated supplies or equipment during the puncture. Keeping extra supplies within reach prevents this disturbing perception.

Precautionary Note !

Keep phlebotomy equipment within reach, but not in a position where it may be disrupted by sudden patient movement. Avoid setting phlebotomy trays on the patient's bed or out of reach.

Precautionary Note !

Case Study
A nurse drawing blood from an emergency department patient had put her supplies out of reach prior to the puncture. After collecting the specimen—and with the needle still in the patient's arm—she had to stretch so far to retrieve the gauze that in the process of reaching she drove the needle deep into the tissue, causing a permanent nerve injury that prevented the patient from returning to work.
Commentary: Even the most skillful phlebotomists can get complacent when performing tasks that have become second nature. Working within one's "comfort zone" still requires an attentiveness to prevent errors in judgement that can drag collectors and those that employ them through a nightmare of legal proceedings.

THE VENIPUNCTURE TECHNIQUE

> *Authors' note: This section assumes a puncture in the antecubital area. Because technique is site-specific, refer to "Alternative Sites" in Chapter 4 for variations in the basic technique specific for draws outside of the antecubital area.*

Procedure

Hyperextending the patient's arm to fully lock the elbow brings the three veins of the antecubital area closer to the surface, making them easier to locate.

1. Select the venipuncture site with consideration for the conditions and restrictions detailed in Chapter 2. Tighten the tourniquet three to four inches above the antecubital area. Make sure the patient's elbow is locked (unless the arm is incapable of hyperextension because of a stroke or other physical condition), so as to bring the veins to the surface of the skin where they can be easily detected. Instruct patients to clench their fist and hold it rather than to pump their hand, which can cause falsely elevated results in some tests (eg, potassium and ionized calcium). Look for the presence of any of the three acceptable veins of the antecubital area, and select the one that provides the most confidence for a successful puncture while considering the inherent risks associated with each vein. (See "Site Selection," Chapter 2.) Choose the median cubital, if available.

    If locating the vein takes an inordinate amount of time, loosen the tourniquet and allow the blood to circulate through the arm prior to the puncture for at least 2 minutes. Leaving a tourniquet on for an extended period of time (longer than 1 minute) results in a condition known as "hemoconcentration," or pooling of the blood below the tourniquet at the intended puncture site. Because this condition can lead to inaccurate results for a wide variety of laboratory tests, tourniquet application beyond 1 minute should be avoided.[2-5,7]

HEMOCONCENTRATION. THE STATIC POOLING OF BLOOD WITHIN THE VEIN AS A RESULT OF PROLONGED TOURNIQUET APPLICATION. AS A RESULT, LARGE MOLECULES (EG, PROTEINS), COAGULATION FACTORS, AND CELLS ACCUMULATE AND, WHEN SAMPLED, WILL YIELD RESULTS THAT DO NOT REFLECT BLOOD LEVELS THAT EXISTED PRIOR TO TOURNIQUET APPLICATION.

Universal Precautions

Defined by the Centers for Disease Control and Prevention (CDC) and OSHA, the term "Universal Precautions" is a method of infection control in which all human blood and certain body fluids are treated as if known to be infectious for HIV, HBV, and other bloodborne pathogens. Practices that reflect universal precautions include:

- Washing hands before and after patient care or if bodily fluids have been handled.
- Wearing gloves whenever contact with body substances, mucous membranes, or nonintact skin is possible.
- Wearing gowns impermeable to liquids when clothing is likely to become soiled or contaminated with body fluids.
- Wearing a mask and protective eyewear or a face shield when the risk of being splashed with body fluids exists.
- Placing intact needle, syringe units, and/or sharps in a designated disposal container as soon as possible without recapping.
- Not breaking or bending needles.
- Refraining from all direct patient care and the handling of patient care equipment if you have a weeping rash.

2. Once a suitable vein has been selected, loosen the tourniquet and assemble the equipment (see Chapter 2).
3. Put on gloves, tighten the tourniquet, and make sure all supplies are within reach. Exercise universal precautions. (See box above.)
4. Locate the vein, and cleanse the site with 70% isopropyl alcohol until clean. If the condition of the patient's arm necessitates excessive cleansing, several alcohol preps may be necessary. Allow the alcohol to dry so that the patient doesn't feel the burning sensation that alcohol can cause when the skin is punctured. Because alcohol dries rapidly, no action may be necessary. (Blowing on the site is not recommended.)

   ☺Third of four secrets of a painless venipuncture! ⟵————

   Once the site has been cleansed, do not contaminate it by repalpating for the vein. If the vein's location has been lost, repalpation can be performed only if the site is cleansed again before puncture.

Often the most prominent vein is palpable but not visible, and it may take more than the allowed 1 minute to relocate after assembling the equipment and retightening the tourniquet. (See "Proper Tourniquet Use" on page 46.) To make relocation quicker, make a mental note of skin markers (moles, skin creases, freckles, etc) on the skin above the vein. After the site has been cleansed and the tourniquet reapplied, these landmarks can prevent the necessity for repalpation, recleansing. and delays in accessing the vein.

Helpful Hint!

5. Perform the puncture. (See illustrations on pages 44-45.)

Using a tube holder

5a. Place the first tube, stopper-end first, into the tube holder without advancing it fully onto the interior needle. Remove the sheath from the needle and set aside for resheathing after the puncture if resheathing is necessary. (See "OSHA's Stance on Needle Recapping and Removal" on page 137.) Grasp the holder placing the thumb on top and two or three fingers underneath as shown. Rest the backs of the fingers firmly on the patient's forearm so that the bevel of the needle faces up and lies just off the skin at the intended puncture site. To keep the open end of the holder accessible for an unhindered exchange of tubes during the draw, grasp the holder at the fingertips, with the wrist turned so that the open end of the holder remains visible and accessible (see Figure 3.1). Inform the patient of the imminent puncture. Be aware that patients have varying degrees of sensitivity and pain tolerance. Do not assume that the patient is prepared for the puncture. A verbal warning of the imminent puncture is appropriate, even if the patient appears unconscious or sedated.

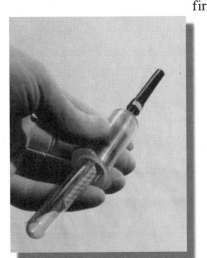

Figure 3.1: Hold tube holders at the tips of fingers make tube exchange easier.

☺Fourth of four secrets of a painless venipuncture!

5b. Stretch the skin by pulling downward on the arm from below the intended puncture site, but not in such a way that it will obstruct the tube holder. When the skin is taut, the needle passes through it much easier and with significantly less sensation. This technique is the single most effective way to minimize the pain of a venipuncture and also anchors the vein to prevent it from rolling away from the needle. With a forward motion, guide the needle into the skin and the vein with a steady advance at an angle of 15 to 30 degrees. Avoid a slow, timid puncture as this will increase the patient's discomfort. Likewise, don't use a rapid, jabbing motion as this will make passing entirely through the vein likely.

5c. Once the needle is anticipated to be within the vein, it is no longer necessary to stretch the skin. With the free hand, loosen the tourniquet (see box: Proper Tourniquet Use, page

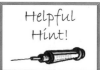

| As the stopper is punctured, overcoming the resistance may displace the needle. To ensure that the needle remains in place when the tube is applied, squeeze the thumb and fingers together gently and cautiously. | Helpful Hint! |

46). Advance the collection tube fully forward so that the interior needle punctures the stopper of the tube. This must be accomplished using the "flanges" or "wings" of the tube holder. If the tube is pushed forward without using these extensions, the pushing pressure may drive the entire assembly forward and advance the needle through the other side of the vein. Therefore, to counteract the pushing pressure exerted on the tube, position the index and middle finger of the free hand on either side of the holder and push the tube onto the needle with the thumb on the bottom of the tube (fig. 3.5). When the thumb and fingers are squeezed together, the tube advances and the stopper is pierced without disturbing the placement of the needle. Allow the tube to fill. The vacuum in the tube will pull blood from the vein and fill the tube to the appropriate level. (See "Minimum Fill Requirements on page 58.)

> Use the flared wings of the tube holder when applying and removing tubes to prevent displacing the needle during collection.

5d. If blood is not obtained, the tube may have lost its vacuum, the needle is improperly positioned in the vein, or the vein is too small for the size of the needle or for a vacuum-assisted draw. Avoid side-to-side manipulation of the needle as an injury can result. Follow the appropriate recovery technique under "Recovering the Failed Venipuncture" on page 56.

5e. After the specimen is collected, removing the blood-filled tube must be done so that while pulling the tube out of the holder, the needle is not pulled out of the vein. To counteract the pulling force exerted on the tube, push against the flared wings of the holder with the thumb or index finger while grasping and pulling the tube (fig.3.7). Gently invert tubes that contain an additive 5 to 10 times as they are removed to prevent coagulation. If more tubes are required, apply and remove subsequent tubes likewise, making sure they are filled in the proper order (see "Order of Draw," page 49). Remove the last tube from the holder before removing the needle to prevent blood from dripping from the tip of the needle.

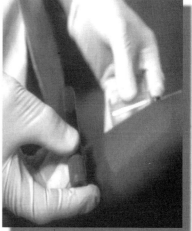

Figure 3.2:Tubes with additives should be inverted 5-10 times immediately after filling.

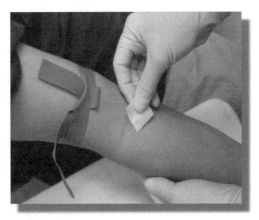

Figure 3.3: Cleanse site with an alcohol prep.

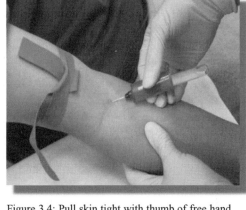

Figure 3.4: Pull skin tight with thumb of free hand and insert needle at a low angle.

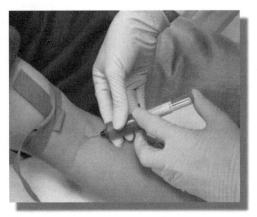

Figure 3.5: Apply tube using flared wings to counteract pushing pressure.

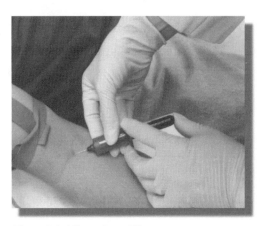

Figure 3.6: Allow tube to fill.

Figure 3.7: Remove tube by pushing against tube holder and invert 5-10 times. Apply and remove additional tubes if necessary according to the order of draw (see page 49).

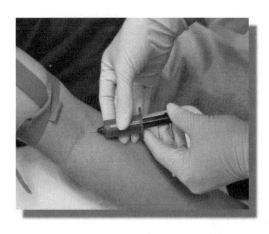

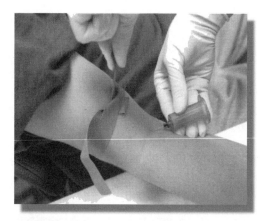

Figure 3.8: Remove last tube and loosen tourniquet.

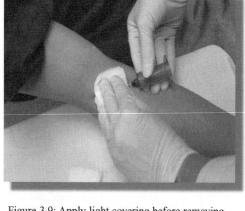

Figure 3.9: Apply light covering before removing needle.

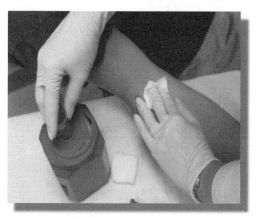

Figure 3.10: Remove needle, apply firm pressure, and conceal and/or dispose of sharp immediately.

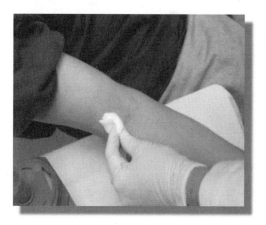

Figure 3.11: Check for bleeding before bandaging.

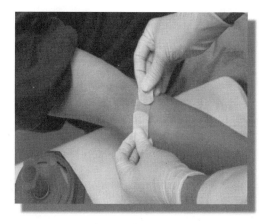

Figure 3.12: Bandage patient.

Proper Tourniquet Use

Studies show that if a tourniquet is left on longer than one minute, results can be altered.[2-5,7] It is preferable, therefore, to release the tourniquet immediately upon accessing the vein.[2] However, if it is anticipated that releasing the tourniquet before all tubes are filled will result in an incomplete collection, the collector must decide which outcome will have the lesser impact on the patient and act accordingly.

To release the tourniquet, pull *downward*, toward the puncture site instead of upward. Pulling in an *upward* direction, toward the patient's shoulder, may result in premature needle withdrawal as the skin surrounding the needle is pulled upward with the tourniquet.

Using a syringe

5a. Unseat the plunger from the barrel by pulling back on it to break the seal, then return the plunger fully forward, expelling all air from the barrel. Remove the sheath and place it within reach for one-handed resheathing if necessary. Grasp the syringe at the fingertips with the thumb on top and two or three fingers underneath as with a tube holder. The plunger must remain accessible so it can be withdrawn without hindrance, and the barrel of the syringe should remain visible throughout the puncture. Rest the backs of the fingers firmly on the patient's forearm so that the bevel of the needle faces up and lies just off the skin at the intended puncture site. Inform the patient of the imminent puncture.

5b. Stretch the skin by pulling downward on the arm from below the intended puncture site, but not in such a way that it will obstruct the syringe. When the skin is taut, the needle passes through it much easier and with significantly less sensation. This reduces pain and anchors the vein to prevent it from rolling away from the needle. With a forward motion, guide the needle into the skin and the vein with a steady advance at an angle of 15 to 30 degrees. A puncture that is too slow and timid will increase the patient's discomfort. Conversely, a rapid, jabbing motion can result in passing through the vein entirely.

Hold the syringe at the tip of the fingers to keep the barrel visible and the plunger accessible.

Helpful Hint!

Do not rely on the flash of blood into the hub of the syringe as an indicator that the vein has been accessed. Under some circumstances a properly positioned needle will not result in a flash of blood into the hub.

Nurses have a tendency to raise the tip of the needle after it enters the skin in an attempt to "pick up" the vein and thread the needle farther as they would in starting an IV. For blood collection, however, all that is necessary is for the bevel to enter the vein. Once it passes through the upper wall of the vein, all forward momentum stops and the needle rests in place while the sample is extracted. Any movement of the needle within the wall of the vein after the vein is accessed is unnecessary.

Helpful Hint!

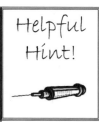

5c. Once the needle is in the vein, it is no longer necessary to stretch the skin. With the free hand, loosen the tourniquet (see box: "Proper Tourniquet Use, page 46"). Pull the plunger back to withdraw the blood. To keep the needle in place during the draw, counteract the pulling force by pushing against the flared wings of the syringe with the thumb or index finger of the same hand. Failure to use these flared wings can cause the needle to withdraw prematurely. Allow the syringe to fill.

5d. If no blood is obtained, the needle may not be positioned properly in the vein. Because side-to-side manipulation of the needle can cause injury, it should be avoided. Moving the needle deeper into the arm should only be attempted if the collector is confident that doing so will not cause injury. A second cause may be that the pulling pressure may be too great and the bevel of the needle may have attached to the upper wall of the vein. Follow the appropriate recovery technique under "Recovering the Failed Venipuncture" on page 56.

> When drawing with a syringe, use the same technique as for tube holders to insert the needle and to maintain placement throughout the collection.

Using winged-infusion (butterfly) sets

5a. If a syringe is coupled to the set, break the seal by pulling back on the plunger to unseat it; then return the plunger fully forward, expelling all air from the barrel. Remove the sheath. Grasp the wings of the set so that the bevel faces up, and squeeze them together with the thumb and index finger. This will allow the other fingers to rest on the patient's forearm and the needle to rest level with the plane of the arm, just above the puncture site. Inform the patient of the imminent puncture.

5b. Stretch the skin by pulling downward on the arm from below the intended puncture site, but not in such a way that it will obstruct the insertion of the needle. This minimizes the pain

Preanalytical Errors

PREANALYTICAL ERRORS—FACTORS INTRODUCED INTO THE SPECIMEN DURING COLLECTION, HANDLING, TRANSPORTATION, OR STORAGE THAT CAN ALTER TEST RESULTS.

It has been estimated that the laboratory provides 70 % of all objective information on health status.[6] Because physicians rely so heavily on laboratory results to diagnose and manage their patients, it is critical that specimens are not alter-ed during collection. Preanalytical errors can cause patients to be misdiagnosed, over- or undermedicated, or otherwise be mismanaged in ways that can be life-threatening. Such errors make up 56% of all specimen result errors.[7] Surprisingly, errors during the testing phase (analytical errors) account for only 13% while errors after the test has been performed (postanalytical errors) constitute 28%. It has been estimated that preanalytical errors cost the average 400-bed hospital $200,000 per year in re-collections and medication errors.[8]

The chart summarizes the types of errors most often overlooked and organizes them into those that occur before, during and after the venipuncture.

It is beyond expectation for every healthcare professional to know and prevent all preanalytical errors. Nursing personnel who are aware of them, however, can keep their impact on patient results to a minimum. For a more thorough discussion of the most common errors committed and the impact they have on the results of the tests collected, refer to Appendix I. It is in the patient's best interest that the principles of specimen collection and preservation—as reflected in the NCCLS standards for blood collection and throughout this book—be understood and observed.

Before Collection	During Collection	After Collection
Patient misidentification	Prolonged tourniquet time	Failure to separate serum from cells
Improper time of collection	Hemolysis	Improper use of serum separators
Wrong tube	Order of Draw	Processing delays
Inadequate fast	Failure to invert tubes	Exposure to light
Prolonged fast	Faulty technique	Improper storage conditions
Exercise	Underfilling tubes	Rimming clots
Patient posture		
Poor coordination with other treatments		
Nonsterile site preparation		
Not coordinating with medication		

Phlebotomy's Best Kept Secret: The Order of Draw

One of the best kept secrets in phlebotomy is the *order of draw*. The order in which the tubes must be filled has been established by NCCLS to avoid cross-contamination of anticoagulants or bacterial contamination of blood cultures.[2]

It is conceivable that the needle used to fill one tube can transfer some of the blood/anticoagulant mixture from that specimen into the next tube filled. The anticoagulants and additives in some tubes can adversely affect results of tests performed on others. For example, lavender-top tubes contain an anticoagulant rich in potassium. If the tube filled after a lavender-top tube is going to be tested for potassium (ie, a red- or green-top tube), any carryover of the blood/anticoagulant mixture from the lavender-top tube to the red- or green-top tube can falsely elevate the potassium level that will be reported, making the patient appear hyperkalemic. It may also add enough potassium to make hypokalemic patients appear normal. Therefore, all lavender-top tubes must be collected *after* red- or green-top tubes. This effect holds true for syringe needles as well as for the inner needle used to puncture the stopper during vacuum-assisted draws.

The order of draw can also impact coagulation studies—for example, protime (PT, also prothrombin time) and partial thromboplastin time (PTT). If the needle transfers a minute amount of anticoagulant from a previous tube into a blue-top tube (used for coagulation studies), the introduction of the foreign anticoagulant can lengthen the protime result and make the patient appear to have a coagulation disorder or to be overmedicated. It can also make an undermedicated patient appear well within therapeutic range. If a blue-top tube is drawn after a tube with a clot activator (some speckled-top tubes), the activator can affect the results of any coagulation studies performed on the blue-top tube. Therefore, blue-top tubes should never be filled *after* a tube that contains an additive. Besides cross-contamination of anticoagulants, violating the order of draw can contaminate blood culture collections. Because the tops of blood collection tubes are not sterile, needles that puncture them are capable of transporting any bacteria they collect from other stoppers into blood culture bottles. The result: the laboratory can report positive blood cultures on patients who are not septic. Such erroneous information can significantly lengthen a patient's stay and result in thousands of dollars of unnecessary tests and medication. Therefore, blood cultures must be collected *before* any other tubes are filled.

The order of draw as established by the NCCLS (Table I) is the same for vacuum-assisted draws as it is for drawing with a syringe. If only two or three tubes are to be collected, fill them as they fall within the recommended order. (A separate order exists for capillary draws. See page 87.)

Table I: The order of draw [2]

1) Tubes or bottles for blood cultures.
2) Red-stopper tubes. All tubes without additives
3) Light-blue stopper tubes. Tubes for coagulation studies. (Contain sodium citrate.)
4) Gel separator tubes. (May contain a clot activator or heparin)
5) Green-stopper tubes. (Contain heparin.)
6) Lavender-stopper tubes. Tubes for hematology and cell counts. (Contain EDTA.)
7) Other tubes (eg, gray stopper, etc.)

NOTE: If drawing only a blue-top tube for special coagulation studies *other than PT or PTT* (eg, factor assays), a discard tube should be drawn first and discarded before the blue-top tube is collected. This prevents contamination by tissue fluids that can enter the tube during the penetration of the needle, and potentially altering the results. NCCLS no longer recommends drawing a discard tube when only a PT or PTT is ordered.

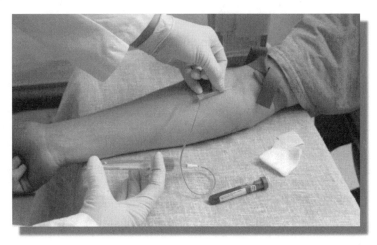

Figure 3.13: Use a tube holder when drawing directly into tubes with a winged infusion set.

Specimen collection with butterfly sets should be performed as with syringes or tube holders in terms of stretching the skin, maintaining a low angle of insertion, and inserting the needle smoothly.

of the puncture and anchors the vein to prevent it from rolling away from the needle. With a forward motion, guide the needle into the skin and the vein with a steady advance, keeping the angle at less than 30 degrees. Slow, timid punctures will increase the patient's discomfort; rapid, jabbing motions will make passing entirely through the vein likely.

5c. Once the needle is anticipated to be in the vein, release the skin. The tourniquet should be released as soon as the vein is accessed to minimize the effects of hemoconcentration (see "Proper Tourniquet Use" on page 46). If using a syringe, pull back on the plunger with gentle pressure using the free hand until a sufficient quantity of blood is obtained. If drawing through a tube holder, push the tubes into the holder and fill in the correct order (see "Order of Draw," page 49), inverting each tube several times as it is removed.

5d. If no blood is obtained while using a syringe, either the needle may not be in the vein or the pulling pressure may be too great and the bevel of the needle has attached to the upper wall of the vein. If no blood is obtained during a vacuum-assisted draw, either the tube has lost its vacuum, the needle is improperly positioned in the vein, or the vein is too small for the needle or for a vacuum-assisted draw. Side-to-side manipulation of the needle can cause injury and should be avoided. Moving the needle deeper into the arm should only be attempted if the collector is confident that doing so will not damage underlying structures. Follow the appropriate recovery technique under "Recovering the Failed Venipuncture" on page 56.

6. Instruct the patient to unclench his/her fist. If the tourniquet is still applied, release it by pulling *downward*, toward the puncture site. This assures that the skin will not pull away from the needle prematurely. Lay 2x2 inch gauze lightly on the insertion point without applying pressure. Remove the needle quickly, and increase pressure on the puncture site. If using a syringe, immediately push the needle through the cap of the first tube to be filled (see "Order of Draw," page 49). Tubes should be standing upright in a tube rack or similar holder and their caps pierced without being held or steadied with the free hand (fig.3.17). Blood should enter down the side of the tube rather than striking the glass bottom of the tube at full force. To remove the needle from a filled tube, grasp the filled tube near the bottom with the free hand and pull the needle from the stopper. Invert tubes with additives several times immediately after filling.

Contaminated needles should be immediately disposed of or resheathed without using the dangerous two-handed recapping method.

For vacuum-assisted draws, the needle should be removed from the arm and placed in a sharps container in one fluid motion. If the needle is engineered for safety, the safety feature should be activated immediately. Any hesitation in disposal or safety-feature activation puts the healthcare professional at risk of an accidental needlestick.

If immediate disposal is not possible, i.e., a bedside sharps container is not available, the needle should be returned to its sheath with a one-handed motion. *Under no circumstances should the needle be recapped with a two-handed recapping method!* (See "Re-using Tube Holders" on page 28, and "OSHA's Stance on Needle Recapping and Removal" on page 137.) On leaving the patient, the contaminated sharp should be immediately discarded in a sharps container. Nursing personnel are best protected, however, when they are supplied with engineered sharps injury protection devices and needle-disposal units at the bedside.

Case Study
A nurse drawing blood from a patient's subclavian central line prepared to fill the tubes from the syringe. Because her facility did not have tube racks available to the nursing staff, she held the tube with one hand and the blood-filled syringe and needle with the other, attempting to puncture the cap as she had done successfully many times before. This time, however, the needle slipped off the cap and punctured her finger. Although she frantically scrubbed the puncture site, a blood test several weeks later revealed that she had acquired hepatitis C.
Commentary: Nurses and nursing personnel should request equipment and supplies be made available that make this tube-filling technique unnecessary.

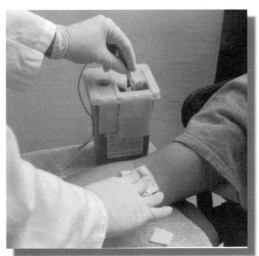

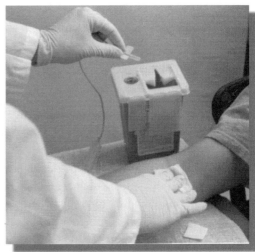

Clockwise from upper left:

Figure 3.14: Discard winged-infusion set immediately upon removal from the patient.

Figure 3.15: If so equipped, activate shielding mechanism on the winged-infusion set immediately after removal from the patient, and discard.

Figure 3.16 Contaminated sharps should be disposed of without hesitation. (See "OSHA's Stance on Needle Recapping and Removal" on page 137.)

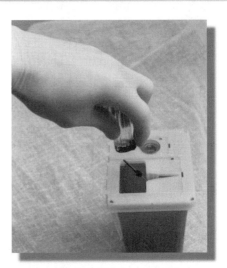

Case Study

A nurse had collected a syringe of blood from a patient while starting an IV. She laid the syringe with its contaminated needle exposed on the bed while taping the IV line. When the patient started kicking, the syringe began to roll off the bed. The nurse instinctively reached for it, and the needle punctured the palm of her hand. She acquired hepatitis C from the exposure.

Commentary: It is imperative that syringes be immediately evacuated and that needles be disposed of without hesitation. The window of vulnerability does not close until the contaminated needle is permanently sheathed or discarded into a sharps container.

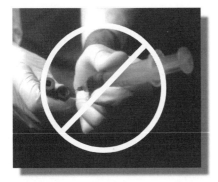

Figure 3.17a: Tubes should **never** be held while filling with a syringe.

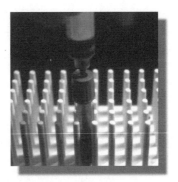

Figure 3.17b: Instead, place tubes in a rack and puncture stoppers with one hand.

7. Maintain several minutes of pressure on the puncture site. It is not always effective to have patients bend their arm up as a substitute for pressure. This technique does not apply adequate pressure on all veins of the antecubital area and should not be trusted.

Collectors must observe the site for bleeding superficially and sucutaneously before bandaging.

Collectors are advised to apply firm pressure until bleeding has stopped. Cooperative patients may be allowed to assist. Complete closure of the puncture site may take several minutes. Remove pressure and watch the insertion point long enough to ensure that the puncture site has sealed. While watching for the site to leak, observe the tissue around the site for any raising or mounding. This could indicate that the skin has sealed, but the puncture in the vein is still open and allowing blood to leak into the surrounding tissue. If you suspect this to be the case, reapply pressure for several more minutes and check again.

Case Study
An outpatient at a small county hospital was drawn in the antecubital area of his left arm for his monthly coagulation studies. Upon completion, the phlebotomist checked the site, saw that there was no visible bleeding, and released the patient. The patient continued to bleed subcutaneously resulting in gradual hemorrhaging into the entire extremity, nearly necessitating its amputation.
Commentary: Collectors may not be aware that their patient is anticoagulant therapy or taking aspirin on a daily basis. Therefore, do not leave a patient or allow a patient to leave your care if you are not certain the puncture has been sealed superficially and subcutaneously.

8. It is imperative that specimens be labeled properly and in the patient's presence. Labeling specimens with abbreviated identifiers to facilitate complete labeling at a later time deviates from the established standards of the procedure and puts patients and nursing personnel and their employers at great risk. Under no circumstances should specimen tubes be labeled *before* they are filled.

Complete labeling includes the following entries:

➢ Patient's first and last names
➢ Unique identification number
➢ Date of collection
➢ Time of collection
➢ Initials of the individual performing the venipuncture.

Preprinted labels may contain the time the specimen is *supposed* to be collected. However, the individual collecting the specimen must make a handwritten entry on the tube and in the permanent records of the *actual* time of collection. This is important for a multitude of tests including blood glucose and therapeutic drug monitoring in which the time of collection is a critical element in the interpretation of the results and in maintaining control over the quality of care.

> Tubes of blood must always be labeled at the bedside with patient identification, the date and time of collection, and the initials of the collector.

Case Study
At a small Midwestern hospital, a lab tech drew a specimen of blood to determine the patient's blood type. She left the room without properly labeling the specimen, drew two more patients, and then returned to the lab to test them all for blood types simultaneously. After being momentarily called away, she returned to her workstation and misidentified the specimens. Because she typed one of the patients incorrectly, a 31-year-old wife and mother of four received incompatible blood and subsequently died.
Commentary: Properly labeling specimens is the most critical step in blood specimen collection. Because improper labeling is potentially fatal, collectors should not allow themselves to leave the patient's side under any circumstances before completely labeling all tubes.

9. Bandage and thank the patient. Discard gloves and other waste in appropriate receptacles. Wash hands, and transport specimens to

The Zero Tolerance Policy for Specimen Labeling Errors ◀━━━ In the Lab

One is hard-pressed to find a laboratory policy that provokes nursing personnel as much as a zero tolerance for receiving unlabeled specimens. To some, rushing unlabeled specimens to the laboratory is perceived as a way to hasten results. However, imposing the burden of specimen identification upon one who did not witness the collection is asking that individual to assume the risk of patient misidentification. As we have seen in the case study on this issue, patients have died as a result of mislabeled specimens. Therefore, few processors or techs in the lab are willing to take that risk if they have not drawn the blood themselves; nor should they. In fact, laboratories have a responsibility to support such resistance in order to preserve the quality of care; and many, if not all, have a zero-tolerance policy for receiving unlabeled or mislabeled specimens.

The standards to which all testing facilities must subscribe support this policy. According to NCCLS, all labels must include the patient's name, date and time of draw, and a patient identification number. In addition, there must also be a way to identify the person who collected the specimen, and tubes must be labeled before leaving the patient's side.[2] Maintaining high standards for specimen collection means upholding this standard and enforcing the policy that any modifications to a specimen label be made only by the individual who labeled the tube initially. If this is not possible, a re-collection should be performed.

Allergies to adhesives

Some patients are allergic to the adhesive in bandages. If the patient indicates such an allergy, an alternative method should be used. Place a sterile 2x2 inch gauze over the puncture site, and apply a gauze wrapping around the circumference of the arm. Make sure the wrap is applied tightly enough to hold the gauze but not so tight so as to restrict circulation. (See "Leaving the patient," page 59.)

the laboratory. If the testing facility is off-site, process and store specimens according to NCCLS standards in regard to the effects of time and temperature on the tests to be performed (see Chapter 6, "Specimen Handling and Storage").

Recovering the Failed Venipuncture

If there is no immediate fill of the tubes or syringe, the collector must then troubleshoot the puncture. There are several conditions that can prevent blood from entering the tube or syringe. These conditions are dependent upon the equipment used.

If using a tube holder

Cause: The tube applied may have lost its vacuum.
Resolution: Apply another tube.

Collapsing veins are usually a result of needle misplacement, excessive vacuum or inappropriate needle selection and cannot always be corrected while still in the vein.

Cause: The needle may not be positioned properly.
Resolution: Pull back on the needle slightly. If flow does not commence, continue to pull back farther until the bevel of the needle is just under the surface of the skin. If this fails, pull the tube within the holder back so that the inner needle no longer punctures the stopper and the vacuum is no longer applied. Re-anchor the vein by pulling the skin down with the thumb of the free hand and move the needle deeper toward the vein. Be careful not to go so deep as to damage underlying structures. Excessive manipulation and side-to-side probing should be avoided.

Cause: The vacuum may be excessive, causing the vein to "collapse" or adhere to the bevel of the needle. This occurs if the diameter of the vein is too small for the vacuum within the tube.
Resolution: Apply a smaller tube of the same type or terminate the puncture and attempt a second puncture using a syringe and a 23-gauge needle with moderate pulling pressure.

If using a syringe

Cause: Excessive pulling pressure on the plunger, forcing the vein to collapse onto the bevel of the needle.

Resolution: Reduce the amount of pulling pressure on the plunger. Minimal pulling pressure can restore the blood flow. If this results in a prolonged draw, however, the specimen may hemolyze or clot within the barrel of the syringe before it can be transferred to tubes and render the specimen unacceptable. To avoid this, complete the draw within 1 minute from the time blood first enters the barrel of the syringe.

Cause: Needle size is too large for the vein.

Resolution: If the needle selected for use is too large for the vein, pulling the plunger may result in the bevel of the needle adhering to the upper wall of the vein. To correct this, pull back on the plunger slowly to apply the least amount of vacuum within the vein. If the specimen enters the syringe too slowly, keep in mind the potential of the specimen to clot within the barrel, as mentioned in the previous scenario. If this technique fails to yield a specimen, discontinue the puncture and repeat, using a smaller needle or a larger vein.

Slow syringe draws can result in clotting in the barrel of the syringe before the collection is over.

Cause: The needle may not be positioned properly.

Resolution: While pulling back on the plunger, slowly withdraw the needle until it is just under the surface of the skin. If the needle originally went through the vein, this will salvage the puncture. If blood does not flow into the syringe, stop short of pulling the needle completely out of the skin and release the plunger so that the force of aspiration is no longer applied. With the bevel of the needle resting just under the skin's surface, re-anchor the vein by pulling the skin down with the thumb of the free hand. Then move the needle deeper toward the vein, being careful not to go so deep as to injure underlying structures. Pull back on the plunger. Excessive manipulation and side-to-side probing should be avoided.

If using a winged-infusion set

The technique for recovering a failed venipuncture while using a butterfly set depends upon the equipment attached to the luer end of the set. If a syringe is attached, follow the recovery instructions under "If using a syringe." Likewise, if a tube holder is attached, refer to the instructions under "If using a tube holder."

Because side-to-side manipulation of the needle is no longer approved by NCCLS, it is even more important to perform the initial puncture accurately, anchor the vein, and maintain the position of the needle.[2] Blindly probing can result in a painful provocation of the underlying nerves or puncture an artery.

Healthcare professionals who are unable to obtain a specimen on two punctures should allow a co-worker to attempt the collection for the sake of the patient. Repeated failures threaten the patient's confidence in the skill and professional judgment of the healthcare professional and generate frustration and anxiety.

> Side to side manipulation of the needle is not recommended and is against the standards for the procedure. Injuries that result from this technique can result in liability.

Minimum Fill Requirements

Blood collection tubes with additives are manufactured with carefully calculated quantities of anticoagulants to ensure that a completely filled tube will be effectively anticoagulated. Underfilling these tubes disrupts the proper blood-to-anticoagulant ratio, which dilutes the specimen, causes excessive anticoagulation, and contributes to erroneous results. All tubes, therefore, should be filled to at least 75% of their stated volume. Blue-top tubes, however, are less forgiving and demand a 90% fill. Because of the nature of the anticoagulant, blue-top tubes filled less than 90% of their stated volume will yield inaccurate PTT results.[9]

Some tubes are designed for use when a low-volume draw is either expected (difficult veins) or necessary (infants, children, or geriatrics) and contain less vacuum and proportionally less anticoagulant. These "pediatric tubes" can be the same size as regular, full-volume tubes, but will not fill to the same level. Some manufacturers place a line on the label of these tubes to approximate their maximum fill level.

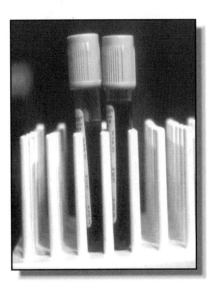

Figure 3.18: Blue top tubes must be filled completely (right). Tubes less than 90 % filled (left) will yield inaccurate PTT results and should be rejected by testing facilities.

The Underfilled Specimen Dilemma ⟵⟶ **In the Lab**

All laboratories within compliance of the standards for laboratory testing uphold strict and well-defined specimen rejection criteria. Among the requirements is that acceptable specimens meet the minimum-fill requirements for tests sensitive to the blood:anticoagulant ratio. When a laboratory receives an underfilled specimen, the processing or analyzing tech is obligated to request a re-collection. The individual responsible for making the decision to reject the specimen is well-aware that his/her request may not be welcome news to the collector, who may be overwhelmed with other patient responsibilities, and that the request may be viewed as an unnecessary interruption. Failing to do so, however, risks reporting inaccurate results and initiating a cascade of events that can interfere with the diagnosis, medication and /or care of the patient. Because laboratories are responsible for the quality of the specimens that it tests, when faced with these two outcomes the testing individual's proper response is to request re-collection and hope that the collector understands that accepting an underfilled specimen puts the patient at risk. Such understanding is at the core of interdepartmental cooperation and is essential for delivering quality care to the patient.

Fortunately, many tests are not dependent upon the tube being completely filled. However, submitting blue-top tubes for PTTs that are not 90 percent filled and other tubes with additives that are not 75 percent filled is requesting that the laboratory compromise its testing integrity.

Leaving the Patient

Healthcare professionals should always be watching for signs that their patients might faint during or after a venipuncture. After assuring that the puncture is sealed and bandaged, observe for signs of vertigo (dizziness) or syncope (fainting). This is especially important for outpatient draws.

Pallor, perspiration, anxiety, light-headedness, hyperventilation, and nausea can preempt a loss of consciousness. Make it a habit to ask patients if they feel all right, but don't rely on their answers totally, especially in the presence of any of the above symptoms. If the patient demonstrates any of these signs, do not attempt to walk the patient to a bed. Refer to the facility's procedure to respond to a patient who faints or loses consciousness. If indicated, lower the patient's head to increase the supply of oxygenated blood to the brain. Ammonia inhalants should be used conservatively as its use can induce an asthma attack if the patient is asthmatic. Call for assistance without leaving the patient's side. If a portable stretcher can be brought into the area, place the patient upon it with assistance. Document the incident. Patients experiencing episodes of vertigo or syncope should be guarded until complete recovery.

Because they are usually recumbent, inpatients rarely experience vertigo or syncope. Nevertheless, observe patients before leaving their side for these symptoms. If the individual was drawn in a sitting position, this observation is even more critical. If the symptoms appear, react as previously described. Request assistance if necessary.

Upon leaving the room of an inpatient, take extra care to return the room to its previous arrangement. If bedside trays, chairs, wastebaskets, bedside rails, and other items were moved, return them for the convenience and safety of the patient. If the patient has to stretch or get out of bed to retrieve an item that has been displaced, a fall or injury could occur. Make no attempt to satisfy a patient's request for water, ambulation, lowering of the bed rails, and the like without making sure that such actions are consistent with the patient's care plan and the physician's orders.

> Collectors can face liability if a patient passes out and sustains an injury during or immediately after a blood draw. Be prepared to protect patients if they exhibit the signs of vertigo or syncope.

Case Study
A patient was brought to a facility's laboratory for blood work by attendants who then left the area. The puncture went smoothly and without incident. As soon as the ambulatory patient left the laboratory area, though, he passed out, falling to the floor and breaking his jaw. The lawsuit that was filed sought damages for the injuries.
Commentary: Recumbent patients rarely experience syncope from blood draws. However, amubulatory patients can pass out with or without warning. Collectors should be on guard for apprehension, anxiety, hyperventilation, pallor, and perspiration, and be prepared to react. Patients with known histories of phlebotomy-induced syncope should be drawn while recumbent and carefully observed before being released.

References

1 Paxton A. Stamping out specimen collection errors. *CAP Today*. May 1999.

2 National Committee for Clinical Laboratory Standards (NCCLS); *Procedures for the Collection of Diagnostic Blood Specimens by Venipuncture*. Approved Standard H3-A4, Villanova, PA; 1998.

3 Becan-McBride K. Preanalytical phase an important requisite of laboratory testing. *Adv Med Lab Professionals*. 1998;10(20):12-17.

4 Narayanan S. The preanalytic phase an important component of laboratory medicine. *Am J Clin Pathol* 2000;113:429-452.

5 Statland B, Bokelund H, Winkel P. Factors contributing to intra-individual variation of serum constituents: 4. Effects of posture and tourniquet application on variation of serum constituents in healthy subjects. *Clin Chem* 1994;20(12):1513-1519.

6 Berger D. Direct-to-consumer testing [Editorial]. *MLO*. 2000;32(3):6.

7 Dale J. Preanalytic Variables in Laboratory Testing. *Lab Med*. 1998;29:540-545.

8 Paxton, A. Stamping out Specimen Collection Errors. *CAP Today*. May 1999.

9 Reneke J, Etzell J, Leslie S, et al. "Prolonged prothrombin time and activated partial thromboplastin time due to underfilled specimen tubes with 109 mmol/L (3.2%) citrate anticoagulant. *Coagulation Transfusion Med*. 1997;109(6):754-757.

Chapter 4

Alternative Sites
Blood Culture Collections
Phlebotomy Liability

VENIPUNCTURES OUTSIDE THE ANTECUBITAL AREA

Outside of the antecubital area, there are a limited number of secondary sites that are acceptable for venipuncture. It is dangerous, however, to assume that any visible vein can be used. Drawing from certain sites without a comprehensive knowledge of superficial anatomy can put the patient at great risk. Healthcare professionals, therefore, must carefully select secondary sites and consider the conditions that may preclude their use.

Hand Veins

The back or posterior side of the hand often offers a network of veins that can be quite prominent and accessible for venipuncture. Bear in mind that hand veins are more delicate and smaller in diameter than the veins of the antecubital fossa. The vacuum within collection tubes is often too great and will collapse the veins of the hands if a vacuum-assisted draw is attempted. Therefore, a syringe or winged-infusion set coupled with a syringe should be used in conjunction with a 22 or 23 gauge needle.

On geriatric patients, hand veins are fragile and can result in *hematoma* formation during the puncture, especially if the tourniquet is applied too tightly. In addition, their platelets are often fewer in number and less functional than those in a younger population.

Therefore, veins do not seal as readily, resulting in *hematoma* formation. If a hematoma forms during the venipuncture, the tourniquet should be released immediately, the needle removed and adequate pressure applied before bandaging. A second attempt may be made on the other hand, if accessible.

HEMATOMA: BRUISING CAUSED BY INFILTRATION OF THE TISSUE BY BLOOD FROM RUPTURED VEINS, ARTERIES, OR CAPILLARIES. DURING VENIPUNCTURES, HEMATOMAS ARE OBSERVED AS RAISING OR MOUNDING OF THE SKIN AT THE PUNCTURE SITE WITH OR WITHOUT IMMEDIATE DISCOLORATION.

The vein on the lateral aspect (thumb side) of the wrist is also an acceptable site for venipuncture. This vein, often used for IV therapy, can be quite prominent. However, because this vein is not firmly anchored, it has a tendency to roll away from the needle when a puncture is attempted. Therefore, it is important to firmly anchor the vein by pulling the skin below the site downward with the thumb of the free hand.

The veins of the anterior (palm side) of the wrist and forearm should never be considered as an alternative site. The network of tendons and nerves serving the hand are precariously close to the surface of the skin. Punctures in this area put the patient at risk of injury.

Veins of the Ankles and Feet

Foot and ankle veins can be acceptable sites for venipunctures in some facilities and on some patients. However, puncturing these veins can result in the formation of clots in patients prone to thrombosis or in tissue necrosis in diabetics. Therefore, before puncturing foot and ankle veins, make sure the facility does not have a policy against such punctures and that the physician has approved of the site. When drawing blood from feet and ankles, avoid vacuum-assisted draws as these veins are generally small in diameter and, therefore, prone to collapse under the excessive pressure of the vacuum. Small-bore needles, 22 or 23 gauge, are recommended.

If unable to obtain blood from the veins of the antecubital area or secondary sites, capillary punctures can yield enough blood if the tests requested can be performed on minute quantities. Often physicians will pare down the test requests to accommodate a capillary puncture if informed of the difficulty in obtaining venous blood. (See "Capillary Punctures," Chapter 5.)

Not all veins are safe to puncture. Collectors must be aware of the acceptable alternative sites.

The veins of the feet and ankles should only be considered with physician approval.

Case Study

At a large northern hospital, a nurse sustained an accidental needlestick while giving a patient an insulin injection. Following the hospital's protocol for the incident, she went to the emergency department (ED) for routine lab work. The ED nurse attempted to collect the specimen from a surface vein on the anterior side of the wrist. Because of careless technique, she drove the needle deep into the tissue and caused a permanent nerve injury. Three surgeries to repair the nerve failed, and the nurse, incapable of lifting more than 10 pounds with the injured arm, is unable to return to acute care nursing.

Commentary: Unorthodox puncture sites can be very unforgiving, especially when the puncture is performed with poor technique.

Case Study

During a routine office visit, the patient's physician ordered his staff to collect a blood specimen. After five unsuccessful attempts to obtain blood, the physician stepped in and attempted a venipuncture on the patient's jugular vein. He missed and sent the patient to the laboratory where her blood was collected on the first attempt in the antecubital area.

Commentary: Fortunately, the patient did not sustain an injury from the failed jugular puncture. If this desperate attempt injured the patient, the physician would have had liability.

Drawing from Vascular Access Devices

Healthcare professionals are often called upon to withdraw blood from vascular access devices such as IV lines, central (intravenous) lines, and arterial lines. The use of these devices is a convenient way to obtain blood specimens without subjecting the patient to a venipuncture. However, such draws are not without risk. Line draws are associated with:

> ➤ Increased likelihood of blood culture contamination
> ➤ Contamination of specimens with IV fluids
> ➤ High rate of hemolysis compared to venipunctures[4]
> ➤ Potential to introduce air embolism into bloodstream
> ➤ Risk of introducing bacteria into bloodstream
> ➤ Risk of line occlusion.

Because these devices offer direct access to the circulatory system, collectors must be highly skilled to minimize these risks.

When collecting blood cultures through vascular access devices, it is difficult to sterilize all potential sources of contamination. Access ports may contain contaminants that cannot be effectively prevented from entering the blood specimen. Additionally, bacteria can colonize deep within indwelling lines and be swept into blood withdrawn for inoculation into blood culture vials. Although careful attention to aseptic technique can reduce contamination rates, to a large degree contamination is an inherent element of blood culture collection from vascular access devices.

To prevent IV fluids from contaminating specimens, collectors must discard calculated volumes of collected blood prior to obtaining an untainted specimen. Because the first blood withdrawn from vascular access devices contains the infusing IV fluids, it is important to calculate the appropriate volume to be discarded according to the device. Each vascular access device has a "dead space volume," which is the volume of fluid that the line contains. To obtain a blood specimen free from the interferences that IV fluids can impart, NCCLS recommends discarding twice the dead space volume for noncoagulation testing and 5 cc of blood or 6 times the dead space volume for coagulation studies. Deviations from these guidelines risk contamination of specimens and erroneous results.

> Because of a high rate of hemolysis and the potential to compromise the specimen with IV fluids, drawing blood from vascular access devices should only be considered if there are no other alternatives.

Specimens drawn through vascular access devices are also typically associated with a high frequency of hemolysis. This characteristic appears to be an inherent quality of vascular access draws rather than of technique, and it is difficult to prevent. Nursing personnel, therefore, are well-advised to avoid line draws, if possible, especially if the delays that come with specimen rejection will interfere with patient care.

Introducing an air embolism into the patient's circulatory system can have tragic results. Because of this and other risks to the patient and the integrity of the specimen, it is imperative that collecting blood through vascular access devices be performed only by nursing professionals trained in the use and maintenance of such devices.

COLLECTING BLOOD CULTURES

Very few blood tests risk the potential for serious consequences to the patient more than an improperly collected blood culture. Bacteria enter the bloodstream (bacteremia) in many ways. In healthy individuals, the body's cellular and immune responses engulf invading organisms before they are allowed to multiply. In acutely ill and immunocompromised patients, however, bacteria can develop into a potentially fatal systemic infection (septicemia). Early detection and treatment rely heavily on blood cultures and the quality with which they are collected.

BACTEREMIA—THE PRESENCE OF BACTERIA IN THE BLOODSTREAM. MAY OR MAY NOT MULTIPLY TO FULMI-
NANT INFECTIONS AND SEPTICEMIA. OFTEN REMOVED BY THE BODY'S CELLULAR AND IMMUNE
RESPONSES IN HEALTHY INDIVIDUALS. CAN DEVELOP INTO LIFE-THREATENING INFECTIONS IN
IMMUNOCOMPROMISED AND ACUTELY OR CHRONICALLY ILL PATIENTS.

SEPTICEMIA—THE PRESENCE OF PATHOGENIC BACTERIA AND THE TOXIC BY-PRODUCTS OF THEIR METABOLISM,
OFTEN PROGRESSING TO A FULMINANT AND LIFE-THREATENING SYSTEMIC INFECTION.

Collectors who are not aware of the important aspects of specimen collection as they pertain to blood cultures can cause positive blood culture results in patients who don't actually have bacteremia. The total cost of this error can be measured in both financial and human terms. Studies show that contaminated blood cultures can increase a patient's hospital stay by 4.5 days and add more than $5000 to the cost of treatment (adjusted for inflation since the study was published).[1,2] More importantly, they can keep patients from rejoining their families and jobs and reclaiming their daily lives.

> Because the concentration of bacteria in blood can be as low as one organism per cc of blood, collecting adequate volumes is critical for capturing circulating bacteria.

Conversely, poor collection practices can yield negative results in patients who actually have bacteremia or septicemia and may lead to life-threatening delays in treatment and, potentially, death. To avoid these errors, collectors must be aware of the importance of aseptic technique and collecting sufficient volumes of blood.

In order to recover organisms that may exist in low concentrations in the bloodstream, it is important to culture large volumes of blood and to do so in several collections. The optimal volume for blood culture collections is considered to be 20 mL of blood per set distributed between two bottles not to exceed 12 cc per vial. *Collecting volumes less than this reduces the potential to recover organisms causing septicemia and risks an unnecessary delay in treatment.*

If drawing both aerobic and anaerobic bottles and the collection yields less than the minimum recommended volume for two bottles, evacuating the maximum recommended volume into the *aerobic* bottle is preferred over dividing lesser amounts between two vials. Most bacteria that cause septicemia are aerobic.

Helpful Hint!

As a means of sampling large volumes, blood cultures are often ordered to be collected in "sets"—pairs of bottles collected at different times and/or from different sites. A "set" consists of *two separate punctures* in which blood is inoculated into two bottles that provide a rich, nutrient growth medium in which all microorganisms known to cause sepsis can multiply to detectable levels. If multiple sets are ordered, it may be appropriate to collect the second set immediately after the first one *if it can be drawn from another site*. The rationale is that in sampling two entirely different bloodstreams, one might increase the chance of capturing organisms that may exist in low concentrations. Otherwise, a 45-minute wait between sets drawn from the same site is recommended.

Helpful Hint!	Many facilities draw two aerobic bottles per set except in patient areas in which anaerobic organisms are frequently encountered, such as obstetric units and surgery floors. In these areas, a set consists of one aerobic bottle and one anaerobic bottle.

Techniques that introduce microorganisms from external sources into culture vials are the bane of every hospital. Positive blood cultures that are inconsistent with legitimate bacteremias fall under the category of "contaminated." Most are tainted because of poor site preparation, but significant portion of these are the result of *transient bacteremias*. Transient bacteremias occur when bacteria enter the bloodstream by stress or trauma to mucous membranes (dental work, injuries to the nasopharyngeal cavities, obstructed bowel, etc) or by invasive procedures that disrupt the integrity of tissue (urinary catheterization, colonoscopy, etc). Typically, they exist momentarily in the bloodstream and then are engulfed by the body's cellular immune response. Because of transient bacteremias and other factors, healthcare facilities have come to accept contamination rates of between 1% and 3% of all blood cultures as impossible to eliminate. But when contamination rates exceed 3%, puncture sites are probably not being cleansed with attention to antiseptic technique. Conducting in-services on site preparation are an effective means of reducing contamination rates to acceptable levels.

Positive blood cultures in patients without symptoms can be a result of transient bacteremia.

How Blood Cultures are Processed   ◄━━━━━━━━━━━━━━◄   **In the Lab**

Upon receipt of a blood culture bottle, the laboratory will immediately aspirate a drop from the bottle, place it on a slide, allow it to dry, perform a Gram's stain and look for organisms under a microscope. The results are recorded (physicians are notified of any positives immediately), and the bottles are then incubated for 5 days (or up to 6 weeks for fungal cultures). Most large hospitals use an automated blood culture incubator that monitors CO_2 levels (a by-product of the growth of microorganisms) within the bottle, sometimes as often as every 10 minutes. When these systems detect a change in the CO_2 concentration, they alert the laboratorian that growth has been detected. The laboratorian will then verify the positive by performing a Gram's stain on a drop of the bottle's contents and looking for microorganisms under a microscope. If present, physicians and/or the nursing staff is notified immediately.

Besides bacteria, CO_2 is also produced by white blood cells (WBCs), albeit in quantities that are too minuscule to alter the environment of a blood culture bottle. However, if more than 12 mL of blood is evacuated into the bottle, the excess WBCs can produce enough CO_2 to trigger the incubator's alarm and force unnecessary confirmatory testing.

Laboratories without automated blood culture equipment inoculate solid media culture plates from the broth immediately upon receipt of the bottles in addition to performing a Gram's stain. Any bacteria in the broth will multiply on the culture plates and become visible colonies after overnight incubation. This "subculturing" is conducted periodically throughout incubation.

Some blood culture systems are so sensitive that one individual microbe alone can multiply during incubation to detectable levels. If that microbe came from the skin because of improper site sterilization, it consumes the same laboratory resources as a legitimately positive culture, although unnecessarily. One study showed that contaminated blood culture can increase the expenditures and overtime hours in a microbiology department by as much as 30 %.[3] Because of the cost of contaminated blood cultures to the laboratory and, subsequently, the facility, it is extremely important that healthcare professionals be mindful of proper site sterilization.

Disinfectants

Iodine-based antiseptics (sometimes used in conjunction with isopropyl alcohol) have become the industry standard for sterilizing puncture sites prior to blood culture collection. Separately packaged alcohol preps and iodine swabs are available, but using them in tandem has been found to be less effective than employing commercially prepared prep kits such as Cepti-Seal® (Medi-Flex® Hospital Products, Overland Park, KS) and Persist™ (BD, Franklin Lakes, NJ).[5]

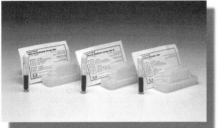

Not all iodine compounds are equal, however. One study showed that iodine tincture is more effective in reducing contamination rates than iodine in an iodophor (eg, povidone).[6] Additionally, iodine tincture has been shown to be more effective than iodine in the form of iodophor solutions *where cultures are not collected by a designated phlebotomy team.* [7]

Figure 4.1: Septi-Ceal® blood culture prep kits contain povidone or tincture iodine. (Photo courtesy of Medi-Flex, Overland Park, Kansas.)

Site Preparation Procedure

Selection of a vein and exercising universal precautions are done in the same way as for any venipuncture. Cleanse the intended puncture site for 1 minute with isopropyl alcohol initially to remove excess surface dirt followed by a 1 minute iodine scrub. The process is completed by placing the iodine swab at the intended point of insertion and moving it outward in circles of increasing diameter until the antiseptic colors the skin 2 inches or more in all directions. Some facilities' procedures call for an initial iodine scrub followed by

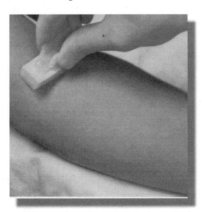
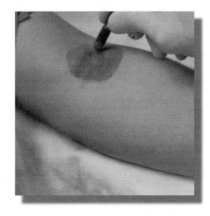

Figure 4.2: Prepare blood culture collection sites with an initial scrub using 70 percent isopropyl alcohol.

Figure 4.3: Complete sterilization by scrubbing with iodine compound and then returning the swab to the center, moving outward in circles of increasing diameter. Iodine must remain on skin for at least 30 seconds to be effective.

cleansing with alcohol and then the final application of iodine in concentric circles of increasing diameter as described. Regardless, the bactericidal effect of iodine is directly proportional to the length of time it is allowed to remain in contact with the skin.

Syringe Draws

Fill the syringe with enough blood to accommodate both aerobic and anaerobic bottles as well as any additional tests that might be ordered. When enough blood has been withdrawn (10-12 cc/bottle), remove the needle from the patient and pierce the stopper of the aerobic bottle. Collectors can monitor fill volumes by making a mark on the bottle's label (volume gradations are usually printed by the manufacturer) to indicate the level at which an appropriate volume of blood will have been added. Upon making the mark, collectors can simply allow the vacuum to pull blood into the broth until the level in the bottle reaches the mark. However, collectors should be attentive as overfilling can lead to false-positive results. (See Precautionary Note, page 73.)

> Collectors can mark culture bottles so the optimum fill volume can be obtained.

If additional blood is collected with a syringe for other lab work, fill the blood culture bottles *first*, and then fill the other lab tubes. If the procedure is reversed, any bacteria that exists on the caps of standard blood collection tubes could be introduced into the blood culture bottles, resulting in a contaminated culture. (See "Order of Draw" on page 49.)

Vacuum-Assisted Draws

For a vacuum-assisted draw, use a winged-infusion set threaded into a standard tube holder. Bottles should never be filled through standard tube holders attached directly to the needle as one would fill other blood collection tubes. When

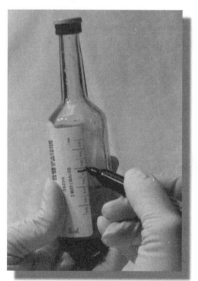

Figure 4.4: Mark blood culture bottles to indicate the appropriate fill volume.

the blood culture bottle is inverted, the potential exists for the nutrient broth to enter the bloodstream. Likewise, the butterfly set should never be used without a tube holder adapter. When not concealed, the needle that punctures the stoppers poses a risk of accidental needlestick. If the blood culture bottle in use does not accommodate the standard tube holder, larger holders are available that fit larger bottles. Check with the manufacturer of the blood culture bottles for availability.

Site Selection: Venipunctures Versus Line Draws

The site from which blood cultures are drawn contributes significantly to the potential for the culture to be contaminated. Draws from vascular access devices (arterial lines, central venous catheters, heparin locks, etc) demonstrate high contamination rates.[4] Because these ports pass through the skin and remain for long periods of time, they are susceptible to bacterial "colonization." Colonized bacteria are those that multiply and accumulate in and around invasive ports but are not necessarily rampant in the bloodstream. Nevertheless, they are easily pulled into blood culture specimens drawn from them. To confirm that a culture is positive because of colonization in the line, a second blood culture must be drawn by venipuncture, and the results compared. (Some facilities have a policy of drawing a peripheral culture at the same time a culture is obtained through a vascular access device.) A negative culture by venipuncture in conjunction with a positive culture by line draw confirms colonization whereas positive cultures drawn from both sites indicate septicemia. However, if the venipuncture culture was contaminated during collection by poor technique, a comparison of the organisms isolated will be necessary to determine if true septicemia exists.

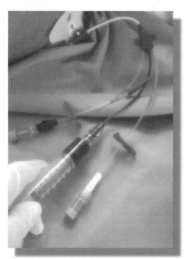

Figure 4.5: Blood cultures collected through a vascular access device have a high rate of contamination and should be avoided if possible.

As you can see, drawing blood cultures from vascular access devices often results in contamination and confirmatory venipunctures that consume valuable hospital resources and, therefore, should be avoided.

! Precautionary Notes for Collecting Blood Cultures !

• *Do not shift your attention from the syringe or bottles while filling.* There is enough vacuum in the bottle to pull more than the recommended fill. If a syringe is used to collect the specimen, the vacuum may pull all the blood from the syringe into the first bottle causing false-positive results from excessive white blood cells. (See "In the Lab: How Blood Cultures Are Processed.")

• *Do not forcefully eject the specimen from the syringe.* If the blood does not evacuate from the syringe, carefully replace the needle with one of a larger bore. *This must be undertaken with extreme caution to protect the collector from an accidental needlestick or exposure to blood.* Withdraw the needle, and repeat for the second bottle.

• *Ensure that air does not enter anaerobic bottles while filling.* Syringes often acquire air bubbles during venipunctures. Minute amounts can compromise an anaerobic environment, killing anaerobic bacteria and, therefore, producing false-negative results.

• *Do not hold the bottle with the free hand positioned near its top when piercing the tops of blood culture bottles with a syringe.* Instead, place bottles on a firm surface and puncture with one hand. Using the free hand to steady the bottle will put the healthcare professional at risk for sustaining an accidental needlestick.

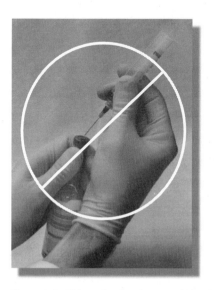 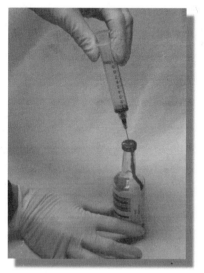

Figure 4.6a: When piercing the tops of blood culture bottles with a syringe, do not hold the bottle with the free hand positioned near its top.

Figure 4.6b: When filled, hold the bottle at its base and remove the needle.

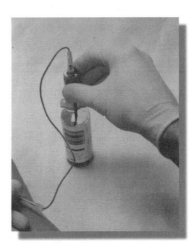

Figure 4.7: Adapters should be used when filling blood culture bottles with winged infusion sets to prevent injury.

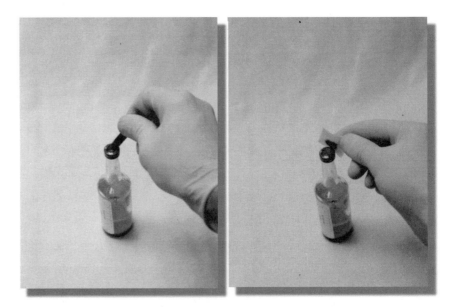

Figure 4.8a&b: Cleansing the top of the blood culture bottle has been shown to reduce the frequency of contamination.[7] Even though the stoppers are sealed and sterilized before shipping, cleansing the bottle before use with alcohol provides additional assurance. Iodine solutions can also be used, but should be allowed to dry and then removed with alcohol. Iodine that remains in contact with the rubber stopper can cause it to deteriorate during the course of incubation, thereby compromising its vacuum and introducing contaminants.

When the vein is accessed, push the tube holder over the neck of the aerobic blood culture bottle to allow the inner needle to puncture the stopper. The vacuum in the bottle will pull the specimen into the broth. Fill to the appropriate volume, and repeat for the anaerobic bottle. Do not overfill. Tubes to be collected for additional lab work should be filled after the blood culture bottles. (See "Order of Draw" on page 49.)

Label the specimens appropriately, bandage the site, and transport the specimens to the testing facility. If other lab work is being collected simultaneously, evacuate blood into blood culture bottles *first*, then fill the other lab tubes according to the NCCLS's recommended order of draw.[8] (See "Order of Draw" on page 49.) To reverse the order is to contaminate the needle.

PHLEBOTOMY LIABILITY

Standard of Care

Healthcare professionals must be aware of the "standard of care" for venipuncture procedures to protect themselves from legal liability that can arise from injuries that result from poor technique. Typically, once a patient hires an attorney to seek compensation for an injury allegedly inflicted during a venipuncture, a standard sequence of events is set into motion to ultimately answer one question: "Did the individual performing the phlebotomy violate the prevailing standard of care for the procedure and/or the facility's policy(ies)?"

If the evidence indicates there may have been some procedural deviations that put the patient at risk, the answer to a second question is sought concurrently: "Did the person responsible for the training and evaluation of the individual performing the venipuncture engage in hiring, training and/or evaluation practices that put the patient at risk?" Attorneys on both sides go to great lengths searching for evidence that will answer these pivotal questions in their favor.

> To establish liability for an injury, it must be established that there was a deviation in the "Standard of Care" for the procedure.

STANDARD OF CARE: THE SEQUENCE OF EVENTS THAT, WHEN FOLLOWED ACCORDING TO THE ESTABLISHED AND ACCEPTED STANDARDS FOR THE PROCEDURE, WILL PREVENT OR MINIMIZE INJURY OR COMPLICATIONS IN THE PROCESS OF ACHIEVING ITS DESIRED OUTCOME.

To establish that a violation of the standard of care for phlebotomy has taken place, attorneys first look for hard evidence that an injury has occurred—evidence that documents an injury has taken place beyond the patient's own claim of pain or complications resulting from the puncture. Unlike whiplash injuries in auto accidents, most phlebotomy-related injuries can be proven or disproved by medical examinations and tests. If a case lacks documented proof that an injury has taken place, the case can still proceed, however. Although from an attorney's perspective, it is easier to pursue a case in which there is documented evidence that an injury has occurred.

If a case is to be pursued, the patient's attorney will research the standard of care for the procedure and for training/evaluation practices. This is accomplished by reviewing the literature, published standards, and the facility's own procedure manual. Authorities on the procedure may also be consulted. Concurrently, the attorney will attempt to reconstruct the sequence of events that led up to the injury through a series of interviews with those involved. These interviews can be informal, private conversations between the attorney and client or formal, recorded question/answer sessions between the attorney and anyone involved in the case by taking a *deposition*. In a deposition, an attorney will ask questions of a witness (patient, phlebotomist, supervisor, etc) and seek to establish a firsthand account of the individual's involvement in the incident that resulted in the injury. This is done under oath and in the presence of a court reporter in an attempt to gather facts and information admissible in court that proves or disproves that there was a deviation in the standard of care.

> Healthcare professionals can be called to provide a *deposition*, which is an account of their involvement in the case.

Throughout the entire process of reconstructing the incident, researching the standard of care, deposing witnesses, and reviewing medical and employment records, each side must act as if it will eventually have to present a convincing case to a jury. If the patient's (plaintiff's) attorney can find convincing evidence that the individual or facility violated the standard of care and by so doing contributed to an injury, hopes are raised that a jury will find the facility liable. Likewise, if the facility's (defense) attorney can convincingly prove that no violations in the standard of care exist, it raises hopes that the jury will exonerate the facility, releasing it from liability. In either case, attorneys must proceed as if the case will come to a trial and that the evidence they uncover will be convincing to a jury. If the case weakens during the process for either side, an out-of-court settlement is usually proposed.

Should the case come to trial, healthcare professionals may be called in to testify about the incident as witnesses. It is important during the trial, as during the deposition, to be aware of the prevailing standard of care and not to testify against it.

Testifying against the literature without extenuating circumstances is futile. If deviations from the standard of care have taken place, they must be justified to the satisfaction of the jury. Using "professional judgment" can be a plausible defense, providing the circumstances were extenuating. Nevertheless, healthcare professionals who are aware of the standard of care for phlebotomy can avoid the embarrassment and anxiety on the witness stand that can ensue when the attorney knows more about the procedure than the witness does.

For those who perform phlebotomy, the only way to avoid the anxiety of depositions and court testimony is to learn to draw a blood specimen according to the standards set forth by the NCCLS, the literature, and the facility's procedure manual and to apply this knowledge every time. A regular review of these documents is important to maintain compliance.

> It is important to know what the Standard of Care is for phlebotomy so that indefensible errors are not committed or defended.

Injuries that Bring Lawsuits

In our experiences reviewing phlebotomy-related lawsuits for attorneys representing either patients or healthcare facilities, we see a recurrence of similar injuries. (In one extreme case however, the phlebotomist was actually implicated in the patient's death.) The injuries patients typically sustain that prompt legal action include:

- ➤ nerve injury
- ➤ hemorrhage from arterial nick
- ➤ hemorrhage from inadequate pressure to the vein
- ➤ complications from drawing from the same side as a mastectomy
- ➤ injuries sustained from syncope during a phlebotomy.

Nerve injuries

Because nerves are neither visible nor palpable, collectors who are unaware of their location in the antecubital area are at risk of injuring them during the collection process. (See illustration of the anatomy of the antecubital area on page 19.) Even though nerve injury is an inherent risk of phlebotomy, almost all such injuries we have seen have been a result of poor technique. However, it is important to know that documentation of a nerve injury alone is not suffi-

Tips on giving a deposition

Depositions are used to set forth admissible evidence that either support or refute accusations of liability. Healthcare professionals who are called upon to give an account of their involvement in an incident that allegedly resulted in an injury should be prepared to respond to probing questions about any and all aspects of their credentials, job responsibilities, involvement in the case, and recollection of the incident. It is best to begin preparing for a deposition as soon as it becomes evident the patient is pursuing legal proceedings. Accusations can take place long after the incident that caused them. Regardless of the time that has passed since the incident took place, healthcare professionals involved should attempt to reconstruct the event through memory and documents that reveal the time and date of the draw, individual performing the puncture, and any other circumstances surrounding the event that can be recalled. It is critical that all speculation be set aside and that one's testimony dwells only upon certainties of the event.

A deposition can be held in any location convenient to all participating parties (a conference room at the facility, an attorney's office, etc.) and typically involves the questioning of only one key witness in the presence of one or both attorneys and a court reporter. It is possible that the patient and/or the facility's risk manager also will be present as observers.

The deposition will begin with the witness taking the oath to tell the truth, followed by introductory remarks by the questioning attorney to define and clarify the process for the witness and establish basic ground rules for answering questions. For the record, the witness will be asked to identify him-/herself and provide a brief personal history. The questioning attorney will then attempt to reconstruct the witness's involvement in the case in an attempt to either capture on record deviations from the standard of care or release the witness from liability, depending

➡➡➡⟶

cient proof that a deviation from the standard of care was made. By performing phlebotomy procedures according to the established and accepted standards, the potential for injury can be minimized, but never eliminated all together. Therefore, an injury alone does not automatically impart liability.

The most common error collectors make that leads to nerve injury is entering the vein at an excessive angle of insertion. When the needle enters the vein acutely, it is much more likely to pass through on the objective of the questioning attorney.

If the questioning is being conducted by the patient's attorney, the facility's attorney should be present to assure that proper procedures are followed and that the questioning attorney doesn't use unethical tactics intimidating lines of questioning, or otherwise offend, confuse, or abuse the witness.

During the course of the deposition, it is critical that the witness maintains composure and answers the questions truthfully and to the best of his/her knowledge. Remember, the answers issued during the deposition become admissible in court. It is best, therefore, not to speculate on the details of the case. Because the deposition can take place months or years after the incident, many facts will simply be forgotten or become vague recollections at best. Avoid temptations to reconstruct the incident based on presumptions, speculation, vague recollections, and assumptions. Questions that attempt to establish a fact about an aspect of the incident with which witnesses are uncertain should be answered with "I don't know," "I don't remember," "I can't respond to that with certainty," etc.

Depositions can be gut-wrenching, especially if the facts that come out establish guilt or reveal deviations from the standard of care. The role of the witness in the deposition is not to exonerate oneself or one's employer, but to uncover the truth. If there have been transgressions from the standard procedure or in training/evaluation practices, they should come to light. Only through pursuit of the truth can justice be served and can a facility benefit from the exposure of lapses in their policies and procedures, thereby preventing future injuries. If there is any indication that the patient suffered an injury during the puncture, healthcare professionals who take the time at the moment to record every aspect of the venipuncture for future reference will save themselves immeasurable anxiety when attempting to reconstruct the events.

the other side of the vein than if entered at a low angle. The "breaking distance" allows the collector a significant margin of error before emerging through the other side of the vein and potentially injuring underlying structures. Another error that often injures nerves is excessive probing in the area of the basilic vein. If it can be shown that collectors had the choice of puncturing the median cubital vein, but chose the basilic vein without justification and subsequently injured the patient, it can be effectively argued that the collector's judgement put the patient at risk. This can bring liability on the

Case Study

In a trial in which a patient was suing the facility for a nerve injury sustained during a venipuncture, the phlebotomist's supervisor testified that a 40-degree angle of insertion was an acceptable angle. Although the patient's attorney cited publication after publication stating a 15- to 30-degree angle of insertion constituted an acceptable angle, the supervisor continued to disagree and testify that an angle beyond that in the published literature was acceptable at their facility. Finally, the attorney read from the laboratory's own procedure manual, which reflected the literature. The supervisor continued to differ.

Commentary: In this trial, the patient's attorney built a convincing case that the facility considered itself immune from the standard of care, even from their own procedures, by supporting an angle of insertion greater than 30 degrees.

facility because many textbooks, including this one, consider the median cubital vein to be the vein of choice. That is not to say that all punctures must be conducted on the median cubital vein, but if this vein can be shown to have been prominent at the time of the puncture, the burden rests on the collector to justify why it was not chosen.

Arterial nicks

> Those who collect blood specimens must observe for the signs of bleeding into the tissue that might occur from arterial nicks or from patients whose veins don't seal readily.

Nicks to the brachial artery are not always evident to the collector in search of a vein. If undetected, hemorrhaging can continue long after the puncture. If blood accumulates in the affected arm, the pressure can result in a compression nerve injury. Collectors must be aware of the signs of an arterial nick, ie, bright red blood with or without rapid hematoma formation, and discontinue the draw immediately. Failure to detect these signs and to apply appropriate pressure to the site puts the patient and facility at risk. If evidence emerges that the signs of an arterial nick were present and the collector failed to react appropriately, the facility may have liability.

The most common errors in technique that involve the brachial artery are an excessive angle of insertion and excessive probing. As discussed under nerve damage, attempts to access the basilic vein must be justified if it can be shown that the median cubital vein was available at the time.

Venous hemorrhage

Collectors should observe puncture site not just for bleeding from the surface puncture, but for bleeding that can occur subcutaneously. Even though the skin may have closed, the vein may continue to bleed into the tissue. Collectors can prevent subcutaneous bleeding by watching the puncture site for a few moments before bandaging to see if a raising or mounding of the tissue occurs and applying additional pressure if necessary. Since it is not always evident which patients have compromised clotting abilities, all patients should be treated as susceptible to subcutaneous bleeding. We know of one case that nearly necessitated amputation of the patient's arm because of an undetected subcutaneous venous bleed after a venipuncture.

Drawing from mastectomy patients

It is beneath the standard of care to draw from the same side as a prior mastectomy by venipuncture or capillary puncture. Because this restriction is so well documented in the standards and literature, attorneys who seek damages to compensate the patient for pain or suffering usually have an easy case. If a draw from the same side as a mastectomy is the only option, the physician should be notified and given the chance to pare down the tests so that enough blood can be obtained by a capillary puncture on the unaffected side. If there are no other options, the physician's permission must be obtained before punctures to the affected side are attempted. Permission should be in writing to appoint the proper liability should the patient subsequently seek damages for pain and suffering that might result.

> Venipunctures on the same side as a mastectomy should never be attempted without the physician's written permission.

Injuries from loss of consciousness

We have seen a number of cases in which patients have sought damages for injuries sustained from passing out either during or shortly after a venipuncture. Arguably, some liability rests on the collector to assure the patient's safety while in his/her care, but how far that liability extends depends on many factors and is best left up to legal experts and juries to decide. Anticipating that every patient has the potential to lose consciousness keeps collectors on alert so that, in the event of syncope, a patient's injuries can be limited or prevented.

Administrative errors

Phlebotomy supervisors, nurse managers, laboratory directors, and human resource managers can all bring liability to their employers for an injury sustained during phlebotomy procedures if it can be shown that the facility engaged in inadequate hiring, training and/or evaluation practices regarding the employee involved in a phlebotomy-related injury. In such cases it can be effectively argued that the facility failed to protect the patient from unskilled employees. The best protection from such liability is to make sure that those involved in the hiring, training and evaluation of collectors in all departments have conservative policies in place that can be put before a judge and jury to prove that adequate measures were implemented and followed for all employees who have blood collection responsibilities.

Policies are great, but without documentation that they were followed, they may as well not exist. Make sure that the policies in your facility regarding hiring, training and evaluation are being followed and that compliance can be proven for all employees.

References

1 Bates DW, Goldman L, Lee TH. Contaminant blood cultures and resource utilization: the true consequences of false-positive results. *JAMA.* 1991; 265:365-369.

2 Schifman R. Phlebotomists at risk. [Editorial]. *Mayo Clin Proc.* 1998;73:703-704.

3 Tiosejo L. Agorrilla J. Results of blood culture contamination study in the emergency room. *Am J Infect Control.* 1998;26(2):170.

4 Garza D, Becan-McBride K. *Phlebotomy Handbook.* 5th ed. Stamford, CT: Appleton & Lange; 1999.

5 Schifman R, Pindur A. The effect of skin disinfection material on reducing blood culture contamination. *Am J Clin Pathol.* 1993;99:536-538.

6 Strand C, Wajsbort R, Sturman K. Effect of iodophor vs tincture skin preparation on blood culture contamination rate. *JAMA.* 1993;269:1004-1006.

7 Schifman R, Strand C, Meier L, et al. Blood culture contamination. *Arch Pathol Lab Med.* 1998;122:216-220.

8 National Committee for Clinical Laboratory Standards. *Procedures for the Collection of Diagnostic Blood Specimens by Venipuncture.* Approved Standard H3-A4, Villanova, P, 1998.

Chapter 5

Capillary Punctures
Pediatric Venipunctures

CAPILLARY PUNCTURES

Specimens collected by venipuncture are preferable over skin (capillary) punctures to ensure quality results. However, if a patient lacks prominent veins and if the tests ordered can be performed on small quantities of blood, a capillary collection may be considered. On newborns, capillary punctures are preferred over venipunctures because of the difficulty in obtaining blood by venipuncture and because of the hazards that venipunctures pose to infants.[1]

Although fingerstick glucose monitoring is the most common application of capillary puncture techniques on adults, technological advancements are making bedside testing on a few drops of blood possible for a growing number of tests. The ability to perform capillary punctures instead of venipunctures minimizes the risk of injury to the patient significantly. Those applications for which capillary punctures may be advantageous include:[1]

> Capillary punctures can be preferable to venipunctures under many circumstances.

- ➤ Severely burned patients
- ➤ Extremely obese patients
- ➤ Patients with thrombotic tendencies
- ➤ Geriatric or other patients in whom superficial veins are either not accessible or very fragile
- ➤ Patients performing tests at home
- ➤ Point-of-care testing
- ➤ Newborn testing
- ➤ Pediatrics and adults with a paralyzing fear of needles.

However, capillary punctures can be more painful than properly performed venipunctures and may lead to erroneous results if improperly performed. To minimize the potential for errors, strict adherence to the principles and techniques of capillary puncture procedures is essential.

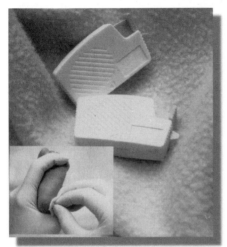

Figure 5.1: Nicky™ heel incision devices. (Photo courtesy of Array Medical, Somerville, NJ).

Equipment

The puncture device should be disposable with a retractable point or blade no longer than 2.0 mm. Punctures deeper than 2.0 mm risk bone penetration. Puncture devices can be spring-loaded or simple lancets for manual penetration. Because devices that necessitate the manual removal of the sharp after use put the collector at risk for an accidental needlestick, facilities should use only those lancets that are immediately retractable.

In addition, capillary punctures are least painful when performed with a spring-loaded device either incorporated into the design or one in which the simple lancet can be loaded into a reusable spring mechanism. If simple lancets are used with a reusable spring device, collectors should employ great care in removing and discarding the contaminated sharp. Manual punctures using simple lancets not in combination with a spring mechanism should be avoided. Other necessary equipment includes alcohol prep pads, gauze pads, gloves, microcollection containers, and a sharps container.

There are two styles of capillary blood collection devices: *incision* devices and *puncture* devices. Incision devices, such as Nicky™ (Helena Laboratories, Beaumont, TX) and Tenderlett® (International Technidyne Corporation, Edison, NJ), cut horizontally across the capillary beds. Puncture devices (lancets) such as QuickHeel® and Microtainer® (both by BD, Franklin Lakes, NJ) and Unistik2® (Owen Mumford, Marietta, GA) penetrate vertically into the tissue. Incision devices have been found to be less traumatic than lancet devices, require fewer repeat incisions, and shorter draw times than lancet devices.[2] For larger volumes, therefore, incision devices have significant advantages over puncture devices. However, for patients who require frequent capillary punctures for tests that

> Many disposable spring-loaded devices are available that operate without exposing the collector to the contaminated sharp.

require minute amounts of blood, for example bedside glucose deter-
minations, puncture devices are advantageous.

Site Selection

The location of the puncture should be carefully considered.
Typically, capillary punctures are performed on the fleshy pad of the
fingertips of patients 12 months of age or older. Fingersticks should
not be performed on the sides of the fingers since the flesh there is
only half as thick as the flesh on the pad, making the risk of piercing
the bone greater.[1] Avoid the use of the thumb, pinky, or index finger.
The skin on the thumb is too thick for adequate penetration while that
of the pinky is not thick enough to ensure that the bone will not be
pierced, which can lead to infection and gangrene; the index finger
should be avoided because it is more sensitive than other fingertips.

For infants up to 12 months, only punctures to the medial or
lateral (inner and outer) plantar surface of either heel are acceptable.
Finger sticks should not be performed on this age group because the
flesh at the fingertips is typically not thick enough to prevent penetration to the bone. While selecting the site for a heelstick, avoid
punctures on excessively bruised or traumatized sites as well as the
back curvature of the heel and the arch where the delicate tendons and
bones are still developing (see figure. 5.4.)

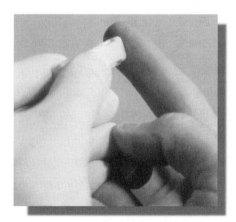

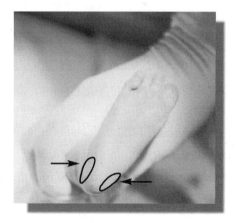

Figure 5.3: NCCLS states that finger sticks
should be performed on the pad of the
fingers instead of the sides since the tissue
on the side of the finger is only half as
thick as that on the pad and therefore less
susceptible to bone penetration.

Figure 5.4: For neonatal patients and infants up
to twelve months, only punctures to
the medial or lateral (inner or outer)
plantar surface of either heel are
acceptable for heelsticks.

! Precautionary Note !

If collecting from an infant's heel, do not force the blood to the puncture site by sliding the finger or thumb along the infant's sole. To do so is to risk damage to the undeveloped tendons of the foot. Instead, force the blood to the puncture site by gently rolling the thumb along the infant's sole from the middle of the foot to the heel.

Procedure

Preparations for the capillary puncture are similar to those for the venipuncture with regard to observing universal precautions, identifying the patient, and preparing the site except that a tourniquet is unnecessary. If the finger or heel is cold to the touch, pre-warming the site for a few minutes with a warm compress or cloth will increase the flow of blood through the capillary beds. Be careful, however, that the temperature of the compress does not exceed 42°C as it may cause burns, especially to neonatal skin. A number of commercial infant heel warmers are available that warm to a limited temperature by a chemical reaction when activated. Either method works well when applied for 3 to 5 minutes prior to the puncture.

Wash hands and put on gloves. Place the puncture device on the cleansed skin with minimum skin compression. Depressing the device forcefully closes the distance between skin and bone, risking bone penetration and the complications that can follow. Release the triggering mechanism of the puncture device, and immediately discard the device if it is not retractable. Wipe away the first drop of blood with gauze to avoid contaminating the specimen with tissue fluid released in the trauma of the puncture. Subsequent drops of blood can then be allowed to freely flow into the collection tube. In the case of a bedside testing device (eg, glucose meter), apply the specimen to the test strip or the appropriate testing interface. It may be necessary to gently squeeze the fingertip or heel to generate a good flow of blood. However, excessive "milking" should not be performed as this technique will likely cause the red cells to rupture (hemolyze) and contaminate the specimen with free hemoglobin and tissue fluid. If excessive squeezing is necessary, the procedure should be terminated and an attempt made on another site after prewarming.

If more than one collection tube is required for testing, follow the proper order of draw established by NCCLS[1]

Order of Draw for Capillary Punctures
1) lavender tubes for blood counts;
2) tubes with other additives;
3) tubes without additives.

Tubes with additives should be periodically mixed during collection with a gentle tap of the finger to prevent coagulation. This technique, however, if excessively employed, can create aerosols to escape from some collection devices. Therefore, proper face protection should be worn. Observe minimum fill requirements for all tubes that contain anticoagulants according to the manufacturer's recommendations.

Once the necessary volume of blood has been collected, discard the retractable puncture device in an approved sharps container, apply pressure with gauze to the puncture site, and cap the collection tube(s). *Before leaving the patient's side*, label the specimens with the patient's name, identification number, date and time of collection, and the initials of the collector as specified in the facility's policy. Bandaging the patient is less critical than for venipunctures and can be left up to the patient. However, neonates and infants should not be bandaged since their skin is much more sensitive to the effects of the adhesive over time and because of the risk of ingestion and/or airway obstruction should the bandage become dislodged. Remove and discard gloves and all supplies and equipment from the area (this is especially important when collecting blood on infants), wash hands, and transport the specimen to the testing facility with consideration given to the effect that time, temperature, and delays in processing will have on test results (see Chapter 6).

> Bandaging capillary punctures can be left up to the adult patient. Newborns, however, should not be bandaged because of the effects of the adhesive on their skin and the risk of ingestion should the bandage become dislodged.

Neonatal Screening
All infants are screened for a battery of metabolic and congenital disorders. Neonatal screening involves applying drops of blood onto absorbent paper and allowing them to dry before transportation to an approved testing facility. Often specimens for neonatal screening are rejected because of inadequate specimen collection. To facilitate accurate results and prevent the trauma of unnecessary re-collections, adhere to the requirements of the testing facility. It is imperative that all the circles of the neonatal screening card are filled from one side of the paper, and completely saturated *on both sides* of the paper. Underfilled circles or cards can result in an inability to perform all the tests required by law.

Table II: Tips on Fingerstick and Heelstick Procedures

<u>Fingerstick</u>

➢ Pre-warm for better blood flow
➢ Puncture on the fleshy pad of the middle or ring finger
➢ Not recommended on newborns
➢ Avoid excessive squeezing of the finger to force blood to flow.

<u>Heelstick</u>

➢ Pre-warm for better blood flow
➢ Puncture on the lateral (outside) or medial (inside) plantar surface of the infant's heel
➢ Not recommended for infants older than 12 months
➢ Do not force blood to the puncture site by rubbing thumb down the length of the infant's sole
➢ Use a retractable incision device that does not penetrate deeper than 2 mm.

> Children have age-specific fears and needs to which collectors should be sensitive.

PEDIATRIC VENIPUNCTURES

Children provide a special challenge to those performing venipunctures and require a different type of compassion than we have for adults. Most of us have an innate fear of the unknown; for children, this fear is especially acute. This section discusses psychological considerations in approaching pediatric patients for venipunctures as well as differences from the procedure as it is performed on adults. Because capillary punctures are far less invasive and can be less traumatic for pediatrics, they should be considered before venipunctures for extremely apprehensive patients. (See the section on "Capillary Punctures" at the beginning of this chapter.)

The psychological needs of children are age-specific. Uneventful venipunctures are in large part a function of the collector's sensitivity and response to those needs. For those performing a child's first venipuncture, the patient should be approached with a great deal of patience and compassion. The effectiveness of one's approach will determine how the child responds to every subsequent venipuncture experience. An uneventful first experience usually makes the next experience considerably easier to bear for the patient and the collector; likewise, a traumatic first experience can make the subsequent event a stressful ordeal for all involved. The attitude, compassion, patience, understanding, and personality of the individual charged with taking the child's first blood test determines, therefore, whether the child will anticipate future blood tests with complacency or anxiety. Investing in a pleasant initial experience makes every subsequent phlebotomy not only less stressful for the patient, but quicker for the healthcare professional to perform.

It also helps to understand that a child can be poorly prepared for a blood test and may have misconceptions about the procedure. Not all parents are skilled at preparing children for the event and may have detailed the procedure in unpleasant terms, or not at all. Parents, siblings, or friends may have talked of traumatic experiences with blood tests so that the child expects all blood tests to be similarly torturous. Because of misconceptions, it is critical that the healthcare professional be perceptive of the child's expectations and level of anxiety from the first moment. It is essential that pediatric patients be given a reasonable amount of time to allay their fears and accept the procedure. Of course, many young patients are well-prepared, but those who are apprehensive deserve an extra measure of patience. For those who have an interest in calming the fears of apprehensive children, a kit of tricks and props called the Phlebotomagician's Pediatric Magic Kit™ (Center for Phlebotomy Education, Ramsey, IN) is available (see Appendix III).

A child's first blood test can have a significant impact on how all future blood tests will be tolerated.

Some pediatric patients will never tolerate having a blood test drawn without putting up a fight. When preparing these patients, it's important to know when enough time has been invested. Extremely difficult patients will be discussed later in this chapter.

Three rules in pediatric phlebotomy should be applied without exception:

1) **Never allow children to see the needle**. Regardless of the size of the needle, the mere sight of sharp steel destined for one's arm is a terrorizing sight for young children and can cause the child to panic. Even if the child appears calm and accepting of the procedure, fear can lurk just beneath the surface of composure and the sight of the needle can be its trigger. If the child insists on seeing the needle, counter with an offer to show the needle only after the procedure is complete.

2) **Never use a needle larger than a 22 gauge on a child.** In fact, a 23 gauge is preferable. Remember that childhood experiences can modify behavior for a lifetime. If that experience is a venipuncture made painful by a large-bore needle, a lifelong phobia is possible. There is no advantage to using a large-bore needle on pediatric patients that justifies the increase in pain that its use can cause.

3) **Always stabilize the child's arm.** It is impossible to be sure that a child will not jump when the needle is inserted. Regardless of the child's appearance of confidence, jerking the arm away from the puncture is a natural reflex that not all children can control. Well-prepared children will anticipate a minor sting when the needle is inserted. However, if the technique results in more-than-expected pain, youngsters may jerk away when the pain exceeds their expected threshold. To prepare for this reflex, having an assistant hold the wrist firmly is good insurance.

Preparing the Pediatric Patient

Pediatric patients who are experienced and comfortable with the procedure are no different to prepare than adult patients. Older children accept this procedure more readily than patients younger than 7 years. For all pediatric patients, however, getting the patient ready begins the moment your eyes meet. Children will be able to detect compassion and tenderness in your face and body language just as you will be able to read anxiety or complacency in theirs. How well you interpret and react to the patient's state of mind determines his/her reaction to this and all subsequent phlebotomies.

> Preparing a child for a blood test begins the moment your eyes meet.

It is beyond the scope of this book to explore nonverbal communication and the psychology of coercion, nor is it necessary since most nursing professionals are receptive and compassionate individuals by nature and dedicated to alleviate suffering. Suffice it to say that for pediatrics, nursing personnel should trust their instincts, yet be prepared to spend the time necessary to calm the fears of those experiencing a venipuncture for the first time.

Because the approach to preparing the pediatric patient for a venipuncture is age-specific, for the purpose of this discussion, we should group pediatrics into three age ranges: birth to twelve months, 1 year to 3 years, 4 years and older.

Age: birth to 12 months

The veins on infants in this age group, especially birth to 6 months, are not well-developed, and those attempting to collect blood should perform capillary punctures unless the physician specifically orders a peripheral specimen. If a peripheral specimen is necessary, the veins of the antecubital area may not be visible or palpable. However, infants usually have well-developed hand veins that can be successfully punctured with careful technique. Regardless of the site, infants have a need for immediate comforting after an experience as traumatic as phlebotomy.

Important Considerations for Neonatal Venipunctures

Site Selection

Veins in neonates are more pronounce on the back side of the hand than in the antecubital area. In addition, it is easier to immobilize the hand of an infant than it is to steady the entire arm, making hand veins the site of choice for neonatal venipunctures. In the absence of prominent hand veins, scalp veins can be an acceptable alternative. However, unless specifically trained to perform punctures on scalp veins, a physician should be consulted.

Positioning the Infant

Venipunctures on newborns must be performed with the assistance of a coworker stabilizing the infant to prevent movement. Minimal restraint is necessary and should not be applied with a force that might cause injury. If a vein on the back of the infant's hand will be attempted, the assistant should curl the infant's hand into a fist to tighten the skin and help anchor the veins.

Tourniquet Use

Collectors or their assistants can grip the infant's wrist or forearm, applying circular pressure to constrict circulation while a hand vein is being located and punctured. Alternatively, a small rubber band can be broken and applied on the forearm as a tourniquet. (Make sure it is removed from the infant's crib or blanket when the procedure is complete!)

Equipment Selection

The use of a syringe attached to a 23 gauge winged-infusion set is often preferred for neonatal venipunctures because of the small diameter of the veins and the maneuverability of the butterfly needle. Assemble the equipment and perform the puncture, being careful not to advance completely through the vein. Because these needles are cut more bluntly than conventional needles, stretching the skin and anchoring the vein is critical to a successful puncture. Once the vein has been accessed (as observed by the flow of blood into the tubing), pull gently on the plunger of the syringe. Excessive pulling pressure will collapse the vein. When enough blood has been collected, terminate the puncture and transfer the specimen to the appropriate collection tubes in compliance with minimum fill requirements. Invert tubes with additives several times to ensure complete anticoagulation.

Volume Considerations

Blood collections on newborns should be carefully monitored with regard to their total blood loss through venipunctures so as not to induce anemia. Limitations apply on single-draw volumes and cumulative volumes based on the weight of the infant (see Table III).

Completing the Procedure

It is imperative that collectors take extra precautions to retrieve all papers, supplies, and equipment from the crib. Small items can be easily ingested and cause suffocation; used sharps can inflict serious injury. A complete accounting of all items used in the area must be performed before leaving the infant.

Table III: Maximum Volumes of Blood to be Drawn From Pediatric Patients

An important aspect of pediatric phlebotomy is to monitor the quantity of blood removed during a venipuncture and during a hospital stay. If the patient is subjected to comprehensive and repeated testing, the risk of iatrogenic anemia (anemia induced through diagnostic testing) can be significant. Limitations to the amount of blood that can be safely withdrawn (listed below) are dependent upon the patient's weight. Should the upper limits of the patient's maximum allowable blood withdrawal be anticipated or reached, conservative measures should be considered to minimize the potential for anemia.

| Patient's Weight | | Maximum amount to be drawn at any one time (mL) | Maximum cumulative amount to be drawn during a hospital stay of 1 month or less (mL) |
lb	kg		
6-8	2.7-3.6	2.5	23
8-10	3.6-4.5	3.5	30
10-25	4.5-6.8	5	40
16-20	7.3-9.1	10	60
21-25	9.5-11.4	10	70
26-30	11.8-13.6	10	80
31-35	14.1-15.9	10	100
36-40	16.4-18.2	10	130
41-45	18.6-20.5	20	140
46-50	20.9-22.7	20	160
51-55	23.2-25.0	20	180
56-60	25.5-27.3	20	200
61-65	27.7-29.5	25	220
66-70	30.0-31.8	30	240
71-75	32.3-34.1	30	250
76-80	34.5-36.4	30	270
81-85	36.8-38.6	30	290
86-90	39.1-40.9	30	310
91-95	41.4-43.2	30	330
96-100	43.6-45.5	30	350

Table from Becan-McBride K. *Textbook of Clinical Laboratory Supervision*, ©1982. Adapted by permission of Prentice Hall, Upper Saddle River, NJ.

Because venipunctures on this age group take a great deal of expertise and advanced phlebotomy technique, they should be performed by those skilled and experienced in neonatal punctures. For that reason, many facilities employ phlebotomy professionals highly skilled in difficult and specialized phlebotomy procedures, such as neonatal venipunctures, throughout the facility. Facilities that assign neonatal venipunctures to nursing personnel should adhere to the established standards for venipuncture procedures (see Chapter 3, "The Venipuncture") and accommodate variations unique to neonatal venipunctures. (See "Important Considerations for Neonatal Venipunctures" box on page 91.) Because of the risk of inducing anemia, it is critical that blood volumes withdrawn be minimal and monitored. (Refer to Table III on page 92.)

Age: 1 to 3 years

Conversationally, there is little that can be done to prepare children in this age group for a venipuncture other than being outwardly pleasant. Outpatients and most inpatients in this group are in the presence of their parent(s) or guardian(s), who can be called upon to hold, comfort, and stabilize the child unless the facility has a policy against soliciting parental assistance. Some parents, however, prefer not to assist or even watch a venipuncture because the pain and distress it may bring to their child is more than they can bear. This apprehension should be recognized and understood. Anxious parents should be allowed to wait outside the room while the collector performs the puncture with the help of a coworker.

> Parents can be instrumental in comforting their child during blood collection procedures. However, anxious parents can heighten the anxiety in their child.

Although the veins of the antecubital area in very young children are well-developed, because of a toddler's inability to remain still, a capillary puncture to the fingertip may be easier to perform, provided the amount of blood required can be obtained by a fingerstick. If a venipuncture is necessary, the use of a 23 gauge needle is essential for a successful puncture and to ensure that the experience is as painless as possible.

Because of the active nature of this age group, gentle physical restraint is necessary to make sure that the arm to be punctured remains immobile during the venipuncture. For outpatients, it is ideal to position the child on the lap of the parent or guardian, who can restrain the free arm of the child while an assistant secures the wrist of the arm to be punctured. For inpatients, or for outpatient situations in which a parent is unable to assist, the patient should lie on a bed or cot with the parent or assistant providing gentle restraint to the free arm and to the wrist of the arm to be punctured. The venipuncture can then be performed as outlined in Chapter 3.

Age: 4 years-adolescents

One of the greatest fears in a child is the fear of the unknown. In the case of a blood test, this fear can often be alleviated in less than 1 minute. Healthcare professionals who read apprehension and anxiety in their pediatric patients should establish a rapport with the child by sitting next to the patient or otherwise getting down to the child's eye level; the effect of a towering, uniformed authority is intimidating enough. Unless already conducted, an introduction is necessary. Ask the patient if this is his/her first blood test. Regardless of the answer, if apprehension is obvious, defuse the child's fear by talking through the procedure step-by-step, speaking in simple terms appropriate to the child's age. To do so, demonstrate the application of the tourniquet by squeezing the child's upper arm where it might be applied to the degree the tourniquet will be tightened. Ask the child to make a fist. Point to the antecubital area, explaining that that's where you will look for a vein. Then explain that you will cleanse the site (for example, "with something cold and kind of smelly") and that you will then ask him/her to look the other way. Explain that, after looking away, he/she will then feel a little "pinch." To give the child an approximation of the sensation, pinch the antecubital area so that the child will know exactly what to expect. Tell the child that, at that point, he/she will be asked to start counting and that you will probably be done by the time he/she gets to 10. Explain that you will then put pressure on the site for a few minutes, you'll bandage it (this is an important selling point: most kids *love* bandages!), and you'll be done.

> Addressing the fear of the unknown in young children is essential to preventing a traumatic experience.

Explaining this procedure takes 1 minute or less. When the child knows what to expect, the fear of the unknown can be put to rest, and the venipuncture has a much greater chance of proceeding without incident.

On younger children in this age group, it is essential that their arms be immobilized during the puncture to prevent unanticipated reactions. The older the child, the more likely the child will accept the procedure without incident. However, collectors should watch for signs of anxiety and apprehension in all age groups and seek the help of an assistant in holding the patient's arm if there is the slightest hint that the patient might not remain still throughout the procedure. Remember, an explosive fear can lurk just beneath the surface of composure.

The secret to applying restraint to a child is not to forcefully restrain a child who appears to be calm or only mildly anxious. Kids don't like to be restrained any more than adults do. A firm, forceful grip often precipitates increased anxiety and the loss of cooperation. It is best, therefore, to use only as much assistance as is necessary to assure the success of the procedure, and no more.

Despite your best efforts to calm an anxious child, some cannot be calmed. Perhaps the fear is so deeply ingrained in them from a prior experience or from someone else's experience or misconception that no degree of compassion will bring the patient to accept the procedure. Should anxiety escalate to a tantrum-like refusal, all hope for an uneventful experience is lost. If the child's parent(s) or guardian(s) are available and willing, their assistance may be necessary to restrain the child so that the procedure can be done quickly and without injury providing it is in keeping with the policies of the facility. If not, coworkers should be asked to assist. *Under no circumstances should a puncture be attempted on an uncooperative child without the assistance necessary to immobilize the intended puncture site and to protect the patient and collector from injury.* No degree of force used to restrain a patient should be so excessive that it could injure the patient. If the patient cannot be restrained without risking injury to the patient or collector, the physician should be notified of the difficulty in obtaining a specimen safely.

> In cases of extreme anxiety, restraining a child may be necessary.

An alternative to venipunctures in extremely anxious patients is to explore the possibility of obtaining the specimen by capillary puncture. This can be an option if the tests requested are minimal and require minute amounts of blood or serum. (See "Capillary Punctures" at the beginning of this chapter.)

Parents can be instrumental or detrimental to the process of drawing blood from their children. If parents show anxiety, the child will take their cue that the procedure is something to be anxious about. Likewise, if parents downplay the significance of the procedure, the child is less likely to be apprehensive. If you sense that the parents can be allies, employ them to become distracters by calling the child's attention away from the procedure. Some parents, however, are so anxious about the procedure that they would rather leave the room than participate. Let them. The presence of an anxious parent can escalate the child's anxiety.

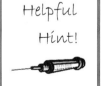

Helpful Hint!

References

1 National Committee for Clinical Laboratory Standards (NCCLS): *Procedures and devices for the collection of diagnostic blood specimens by skin puncture.* Approved Standard H4-A4, Villanova, PA:1999.
2 Matthews D. Comparative studies of time requirement and repeat sticks during heelstick. *Neonatal Int Care.*May/June, 1992;66-68.

Chapter 6

Specimen Handling and Storage

Authors' Note: The list of handling, storage, and transportation requirements for every lab test is extensive and beyond the scope of this text. The information presented here is intended to provide general handling, storage, and transportation guidelines for blood specimens to be tested in a clinical laboratory. Because there are no rules of specimen transportation and storage that can be universally applied to all tubes for all tests all of the time, those collecting blood specimens should consult their testing laboratory for any specific requirements relating to the analyte to be tested.

Although specimen collection is critical, the influence the blood collector has on results doesn't end when the blood fills the tube. Any number of errors that can be introduced into the specimen during its handling, storage, and transportation can significantly alter the results. If healthcare professionals don't avoid these errors, inaccurate results can result and have a life-threatening impact on a patient's diagnosis, treatment, and management.

Some of the most common preanalytical errors and the effects they can have on specimen results are summarized in Appendix I.

GENERAL REQUIREMENTS

Handling

From the moment the blood enters the tube, its cellular and chemical components are subject to the effects of time, temperature, light, and two natural processes that take place when blood is no longer in circulation: clot formation and the exchange of analytes between cells and *serum* or *plasma*. Disregarding these effects can introduce preanalytical errors (see box, page 48) into the specimen within hours of collection.

A common preanalytical error is to allow clotting to take place in a specimen for which clotting is not intended. Clotting can occur during a vacuum-assisted draw if tubes that contain anticoagulants are not inverted 5 to 10 times immediately after collection. Specimens drawn with syringes are especially vulnerable to clotting and require special consideration. The moment blood enters the barrel of the syringe, the clotting process begins. If the needle is not positioned correctly in the vein and blood merely trickles into the syringe, it may take a considerable amount of time to collect the specimen and transfer it into the tubes. If this time exceeds 1 minute, significant clotting may take place. Not only will clotting make it difficult to evacuate the specimen, but if the clots are small enough to go undetected they can alter the results without notice.

> Syringes should be evacuated into tubes as soon as possible after the puncture is complete.

Case Study

At a large university-based hospital, a combative patient came to the emergency department (ED). The nurse drew blood specimens and sent them to the laboratory. Testing revealed a hemoglobin result of 5.6. The patient demonstrated no clinical signs of anemia or acute blood loss. Nevertheless, the ED team was forced to react with a flurry of activity and further testing. Having found no other evidence to support such a low hemoglobin, another CBC was ordered, which revealed a hemoglobin of 13.6.

Commentary: In this case, it was learned that the 5.6 hemoglobin result was due to a preanalytical error. The ED nurse had collected the specimen in a syringe while starting an IV on the patient, which is an acceptable practice. However, after filling the syringe, he had set it aside and tended to the IV fluids. Some time later, the syringe was evacuated into the tubes and sent to the lab. In the time the blood sat in the syringe, significant clotting had likely occurred, but not enough to become detectable or to interfere with evacuating a portion of the specimen into the CBC tube. Because many cells had been bound up in the clot, the aliquot of specimen evacuated into the tube no longer represented the concentration of RBCs in vivo and, therefore, misrepresented the patient's actual hemoglobin concentration.

Whether using a syringe or a tube holder, without an *immediate* inversion of tubes that contain anticoagulants, partial or complete clotting can occur. When performing a vacuum-assisted draw, 5 to10 gentle inversions of the tube immediately after filling are sufficient. Avoid shaking the tubes vigorously as this can result in hemolysis. If not inverted immediately upon filling, invert the tubes as soon as the venipuncture has been completed.

ANALYTES—COMPONENTS OF BLOOD THAT ARE TESTED BY A CLINICAL LABORATORY
PLASMA—THE LIQUID PORTION OF THE BLOOD AFTER CENTRIFUGATION OF A SPECIMEN IN WHICH AN ANTICOAGULANT HAS PREVENTED CLOT FORMATION.
SERUM—THE LIQUID PORTION OF THE BLOOD AFTER CENTRIFUGATION OF A SPECIMEN THAT IS ALLOWED TO CLOT (RED-TOP TUBES).

Storage and Transportation Conditions

To prevent sample deterioration, proper storage and transportation conditions of the specimen must be maintained if delayed testing is anticipated. Specimens collected in long-term care facilities, physicians' offices, and other sites remote from the testing facility are particularly vulnerable to the deteriorating effects that time, temperature, and light can have on the ultimate results. If these factors take effect, the impact on the patient can be in the form of missed or incorrect diagnosis, over- or undermedication, and ineffective patient management.

Effects of serum/cell contact

The chemical composition of a blood specimen can change dramatical when it is allowed to sit with the serum/plasma remaining in contact with the cells. Therefore, removing serum/plasma from the

> **! Precautionary Note !**
> Healthcare professionals who process specimens by centrifugation and separation of serum or plasma into transport tubes should exercise universal precautions, according to the OSHA Bloodborne Pathogen Standard.(See box, page 41).

Table IV: Analytes in serum or plasma that change over time when exposed to cells:[1-3]

Falsely elevated	Falsely decreased
• Lactate dehydrogenase (LD)	• Glucose
• Phosphorous (PO4$^+$)	• Ionized calcium (Ca^{++})
• Ammonia (NH4$^-$)	• Bicarbonate (CO_2)
• Potassium (K$^+$)	• Folate
• Creatinine	
• B-12	
• ALT	
• AST	

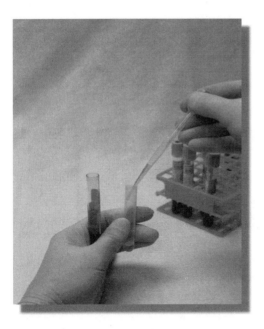

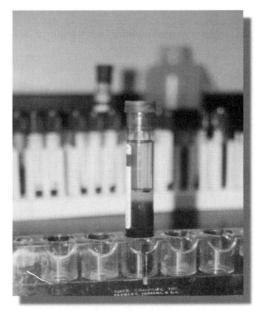

Figure 6.1: Separating the serum/plasma from the cells can be done by removing the stopper, and transferring an aliquot to a transfer tube with a transfer pipet.

Figure 6.2: Some specimen tubes contain a serum separating gel designed to separate serum or plasma from the cells during centrifugation negating the need to physically access the specimen.

Helpful Hint!

If processing specimens for transportation to testing facilities remote to the drawing site, nonadditive plastic transfer tubes with caps should be available from the testing laboratory for transferring serum.

cells within 2 hours of collection is critical for preserving the concentration of many *analytes*.

Centrifugation forces all the cellular components of the blood (red cells, white cells, and platelets) to the bottom of the tube with the cell-free serum to be tested remaining at the top of the tube. Before separation, tubes without anticoagulants should be allowed to sit for 30 minutes for complete clotting to take place. (Tubes with a clot activator still require at least 30 minutes for complete clotting to occur.) Tubes with anticoagulants can be centrifuged immediately. After centrifugation, separating the serum/plasma from the cells can be done by removing the stopper, and transferring an aliquot to a transfer tube with a dropper (transfer pipet). Any spills should be immediately cleaned up. (See Chapter 8, "Practices and Products for Exposure Prevention.")

Table V: Analytes affected by storage in gel-separator tubes [2, 4]	
Therapeutic Drugs*	Other testing
Phenytoin (Dilantin®**)	Tricyclic antidepressants
Phenobarbital	(amitriptyline, imipramine,
Quinidine	etc.)
Carbamazepine (Tegretol®✝)	Progesterone
Lidocaine	Blood bank testing

*Gel-separator tubes from some manufacturers do not affect any/all therapeutic drugs listed. Consult package inserts accompanying gel-separator tubes for brand-specific limitations.
**Dilantin® is a registered trademark of Parke-Davis (Morris Plains, NJ)
✝Tegretol® is a registered trademark of Novartis Pharmaceuticals Corp. (East Hanover, NJ)

To facilitate processing, some specimen tubes contain a serum-separating gel designed to separate serum or plasma from the cells during centrifugation, negating the need to physically access the specimen. This gel positions itself between the serum/plasma and cells during centrifugation and serves as an effective barrier to prevent ions and compounds from changing in their concentration. When stored under proper conditions, serum or plasma can be exposed to the gel barrier for 2 to 5 days.

The FDA has approved the gel tubes of some manufacturers for all analytes while those of other manufacturers have been shown to affect the results of some therapeutic drugs. Therefore, it is prudent to avoid collecting any therapeutic drug tests into gel-separator tubes unless confirmed by the testing laboratory that the tube is appropriate. Table V lists some of the analytes that can be affected when stored in a gel-separator tube.

> Specimens collected for bilirubin should be protected from light immediately after collection.

Effects of light

Some analytes also deteriorate when exposed to light. The most commonly encountered light-sensitive analyte is bilirubin, which has been shown to undergo up to a 50 % reduction in concentration when exposed to light for 1 hour.[5] Other light-sensitive analytes include carotene, RBC folate and Vitamin B[12]. When testing for this constituent, the specimen can be shielded from light during handling, storage, and transportation by transferring the serum or plasma into a brown or light-restrictive transport tube or by wrapping the specimen in aluminum foil or encasing in a light-tight transport canister.

Red-top tubes should be centrifuged and the serum removed from contact with the red cells within two hours of collection.

! Precautionary
Note !
Refrigerating clotted specimens, even for short periods of time, without separating the serum from the cells is unacceptable when testing includes potassium. Under refrigerated conditions, potassium leaks from the cells into the serum/plasma resulting in falsely elevated results.

SITE-DEPENDENT REQUIREMENTS

To put the body of knowledge on specimen preservation in a nursing perspective, this section organizes the effects of time, temperature, and light according to the proximity of the testing facility and tube type. All these effects are well-documented and should be reflected in the storage and transportation practices of all testing facilities. Although some aspects of specimen management are subject to variables unique to the relationship between the lab and the collection site, the general precepts of specimen preservation mentioned here are those that collectors should find to be universally applied.

On-Site Testing Facilities

In hospitals, physician office labs (POLs), and other settings in which the testing facility is on-site and specimens can be processed within 2 hours, specimens should be transported to the laboratory or testing area immediately. If transportation or processing is expected to be delayed beyond 2 hours after specimen collection, refer to the handling, storage, and transportation recommendations detailed in "Off-Site Testing Facilities."

Lavender-top tubes

Tubes collected for hematological studies (CBC, reticulocytes, sedimentation rate, platelet count, etc) may be transported to the laboratory testing area at room temperature. Refrigerate specimens for sedimentation rates (sed rates, Westergren Sedimentation Rates, WSR, ESR, etc) if testing is not anticipated to proceed within 4 hours. Some analytes unstable at room temperature are required to be drawn in lavender-top tubes. When collection requirements suggest immediate chilling, specimens should be transported on ice or in ice water immediately after collection and labeling.

Red-top/speckled-top (gel) tubes

Serum or plasma remaining in contact with red blood cells undergo significant and rapid changes (see Table IV). Refrigerated temperatures accelerate some of these biochemical changes. Unless evidence exists that the tests to be performed are not affected by serum/cell contact, specimens collected in red-top or speckled-top (gel) tubes should be transported to the laboratory or testing facility at room temperature within 2 hours.

If processing and separation are to be delayed beyond 2 hours, the specimens should be centrifuged and the serum separated from the cells. For many tests, separated serum is stable at room temperature up to 8 hours after collection. However, unless the testing facility requires separated serum/plasma to remain at room temperature, refrigerating separated serum/plasma ensures the stability of the specimen.

Some tests require that the serum be immediately refrigerated between 2 and 5^{0}C (see Table VI).

Table VI[2,3]
Analytes that are unstable at room temperature
(irrespective of contact with cells)

➢ Ammonia
➢ Acid phosphatase (ACP)
➢ Coagulation studies (PT* fibrinogen, factor assays, etc)
➢ Ethanol*
➢ Gastrin
➢ Lactic acid
➢ Parathyroid hormone (PTH)
➢ Renin

*after tube is opened

Green-top tubes

In general, follow the same guidelines for the handling, storage, and transportation of green-top tubes as you would for red-top tubes. Unless whole blood will be tested, separate the plasma from the cells within 2 hours and do not refrigerate in the interim. Some tests collected in green-top tubes, however, require that the specimen undergo immediate chilling (see Table VI). If these tests are ordered in addition to potassium, collect a separate tube for the potassium, keep it at room temperature, and separate the plasma from the cells within 2 hours.

If there is any question, consult the testing facility for specific handling, storage, and transportation requirements with regard to the test in question.

! Precautionary Note !

Green-top tubes contain heparin in combination with either ammonia, sodium, or lithium. It is important that when testing for ammonia, the green-top tube used does not contain the ammonia heparin additive. Likewise, when collecting for lithium, the required green-top tube must not contain the lithium heparin additive.

Blue-top tubes

Some clotting factors in the blood deteriorate rapidly once collected. Because blue-top tubes are used to test for such factors, they should be processed as soon as possible. Even though a pro-thrombin time (PT) is stable in an uncentrifuged, unrefrigerated tube for up to 24 hours, a partial thromboplastin time (PTT) deteriorates significantly after 4 hours regardless of the storage and/or transportation temperature.[6,7] If testing is delayed beyond 4 hours, PTT results will be unreliable.

Because of their instability, PTT and some factor assays per-formed and reported on blue-top tubes that are not processed and tested within 4 hours of collection can present misleading informa-tion about the patient's clotting ability and/or anticoagulant dosage. If coagulation tests are not performed with strict compliance to the lim-itations of time and temperature, the result can be over- or under-medication of the patient, which risks stroke, hemorrhage, or death.

Off-Site Testing Facilities

Lavender-top tubes

If testing cannot be performed immediately, lavender-top tubes collected for hematological studies (CBC, hemoglobin/hemat-ocrit, platelet counts, WBC counts, reticulocyte counts, etc) should be stored and transported under refrigerated conditions. Once refrigerat-ed, cell counts are stable up to 24 hours. If the lavender-top tube is being collected for a sedimentation rate (SR, ESR, or WSR), testing should begin within 4 hours if the specimen is kept at room tempera-ture. Refrigeration extends this limitation to 12 hours. Since these tests require *whole blood*, lavender-top tubes should not be cen-trifuged.

> *WHOLE BLOOD*—BLOOD IN WHICH COAGULATION IS INHIBITED BY THE ACTIV-ITY OF ANTICOAGULANTS AND THE CELLULAR MATERIAL IS ALLOWED TO REMAIN IN SUSPENSION WITH THE PLASMA. UNCENTRIFUGED ANTICOAGULATED BLOOD.

Red-top/speckled (gel) tubes

As mentioned, the concentration of many analytes changes significantly when exposed to RBCs for prolonged periods of time (see Table IV). When anticipating delays in testing beyond 2 hours, allow 20 to 30 minutes for complete clotting (at room temperature) to take place, then centrifuge the specimen at the speed and time estab-lished by the testing facility. Serum must be removed from the RBCs

Why do some tests take so long? ◄————◄ In the Lab

There are many variables in clinical laboratory testing that affect the lab's ability to put out results in a timely manner. Staffing shortages, equipment malfunctions, missing specimens and orders, unverifiable results, communication snafus, and many other avoidable and unavoidable events can bring the testing and reporting process to a screeching halt. Most laboratories, however, have contingency plans to accommodate the more frequent and predictable delays. Implementing backup processes can be tedious and invariably delays result reporting. From a nursing standpoint, patience with such interruptions in service is often difficult, but always prudent.

Other delays, though, are an inherent element of clinical laboratory testing and cannot be hastened. Two of the most frequent legitimate delays are associated with "timed tests" and "send-outs." Timed tests are those that require a fixed amount of time to render results. Not all tests provide instantaneous results. Some incorporate incubation phases while others require the serum to undergo a time-consuming pretreatment step to eliminate interfering factors. Although robotics and computerized automation continue to shorten the "turnaround time" for lab tests, some functions simply cannot be shortened. For example, blood cultures cannot be finalized as negative until they are allowed to incubate for 5 days. Although preliminary reports are issued, it is unreasonable to expect the first preliminary result until the culture has been allowed to incubate at least 12 hours.

Bacteria need at least that much time to multiply to detectable levels. Immediate Gram's stains of the specimen, however, are usually performed within minutes and can serve as a preliminary result.

Sedimentation rates measure how far RBCs will settle in 1 hour when mixed with saline and placed upright in a column. In certain disease states and inflammation, they fall quite rapidly. Because the results are measured in millimeters per hour, it takes an hour of settling to make the determination. Some manufacturers are successfully modifying the procedure so that sed rate results don't take so long to obtain. However in most facilities, the testing phase of sed rates cannot be hastened by ordering them as "stat."

All laboratories have to rely to some extent on reference labs to perform those tests for which a low volume of orders makes it impractical to perform in-house. There are well over 1000 tests that can be performed on blood; no laboratory can do them all. Every testing facility, therefore, has its own list of "send-outs." Depending on the test ordered, the reference lab with which the on-site testing facility contracts to perform infrequently ordered or "esoteric" tests can be across the street, across town, or across the country. Naturally, the farther away the reference lab is, the longer it will take to obtain results. Fortunately, the results of such esoteric tests are usually not needed immediately, yet they provide important information to assist in the diagnosis and long-term management of the patient.

preferably within 1 hour, but no longer than 2 hours after collection and stored according to the test requirements.[2] This separation can be accomplished by transferring the serum or plasma into a separate transfer tube or, in the case of a gel-separator tube, centrifugation.

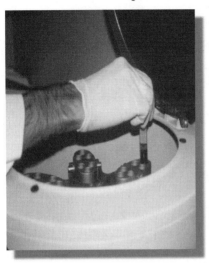

Separated serum can be stored at room temperature for up to 8 hours without compromising the stability of most analytes.[2] However, some analytes deteriorate rapidly at room temperature (see Table VI). If these and other temperature-sensitive analytes are to be tested at an off-site testing facility and a delay in transportation and/or testing is anticipated, immediate processing is essential to provide accurate results. Centrifugation should begin *immediately after complete clotting has taken place* for red-top tubes. After centrifugation, the serum should be separated within 2 hours and refrigerated pending transportation to the testing facility.

Figure 6.3: Serum separation can be accomplished by the use of a gel separator tube and centrifugation.

Some testing sites request temperature-sensitive analytes to be transported without centrifugation and separation. For these analytes it is critical that the specimen remains in contact with ice chips or an ice bath as opposed to simple refrigeration. This can be accomplished with leak-proof bags or containers designed specifically for transporting such specimens and ensure the analyte being tested will be optimally preserved.

Whenever potassium is ordered in conjunction with analytes that need to be preserved at low temperatures, a separate tube should be collected for the potassium.

! Precautionary Note !
Gel-barrier tubes are not appropriate for all analytes. Refer to Table V, page 101.

Green-top tubes

Whole blood specimens in green-top tubes are not to be chilled while awaiting transportation to the testing facility unless it is documented that immediate chilling is necessary to preserve values (see Table VI).[2] For these, qualifying specimens should be cooled immediately by placing the specimen in a container of crushed ice or ice water after it is collected and labeled. As with red-top tubes, when collecting specimens for potassium in conjunction with tests that require specimens to be stored at cold temperatures without separation from the cells, a second tube should be collected for the potassium. For most other analytes, processing requirements on green-top tubes are the same as for red-top tubes.

Blue-top tubes

The plasma from blue-top tubes can be tested for a PT, PTT, and other coagulation factors. Since many clotting factors deteriorate within hours of collection, it is critical that these tubes be processed and tested within 4 hours of collection. PT results can be reliable in an unrefrigerated, uncentrifuged specimen for up to 24 hours after collection. However, PTTs are less forgiving and deteriorate after 4 hours, regardless of temperature or storage conditions. The difference in PTT results from improper storage and delayed testing on a blue-top tube is significant and could impact the way in which the physician decides to medicate the patient. If the medication is based on erroneous results generated from a specimen that was improperly handled and processed, those involved in the specimen handling have put the patient at risk.

Summary

To summarize, despite the variety of optimum conditions for individual analytes, adherence to basic specimen-handling guidelines will preserve specimen integrity in the majority of cases. Keeping in mind that there are exceptions, general guidelines can be summarized as follows:

> ➢ If specimen testing on serum or plasma is to be delayed beyond 2 hours, the serum or plasma should be separated from the cells by centrifugation and removed from contact with RBCs.

> ➢ If the specimen was collected in a gel-separator tube, centrifugation alone will accomplish serum separation, provided complete clotting has been allowed to occur.

> ➢ Tubes with gel separators should not be used on tricyclic antidepressants, progesterone, and many therapeutic drugs. However, affected tests depend on the tube's manufacturer. The testing facility should be aware of the limitations of the tubes in use.

> ➢ If the tube does not contain a gel separator, the serum/plasma should be removed from the cells within 2 hours of centrifugation, placed into a separate transfer tube, and stored at the appropriate temperature according to the test criteria.

! Precautionary Note !

If processing specimens requires centrifugation or the transfer of serum or plasma into transfer tubes, use appropriate personal protection devices (gloves, gown, face shield, etc) and follow universal precautions according to the OSHA Bloodborne Pathogen Standard.

> ➢ If the test ordered is for PTT, the blue-top tube should be tested within 4 hours of collection.
>
> ➢ If the test ordered is for a CBC or other hematological studies, the uncentrifuged lavender-top specimen should be refrigerated if testing is to be delayed longer than 4 hours.

Because the storage temperature of the separated serum or plasma is dependent upon the analyte being tested, the entire battery of tests ordered must be considered when determining proper storage and transportation temperatures and conditions, and they should be accommodated accordingly. Whenever the tests ordered require different storage conditions, drawing extra tubes or dividing the serum/plasma into separate fractions may be necessary so that all blood values can be appropriately preserved. The testing facility should provide drawing stations with a desk reference containing specific information on storage and handling for each test.

Authors' Note

Despite efforts to monitor and regulate compliance with established laboratory standards, lax adherence to the effects of time and temperature during storage and handling persists. Those collecting blood specimens must be aware of the time limitations and environmental extremes to which some analytes are sensitive in order to ensure the integrity of the specimen and, therefore, the accuracy of the result. If a testing facility accepts and tests specimens collected, handled, stored, and transported outside of the standards as established by NCCLS and set forth in the literature, such deviations should be questioned and justified.

References

1 Dale J. Preanalytical variables in laboratory testing. *Lab Med*. 1998; 29:540-545.

2 National Committee for Clinical Laboratory Standards. *Procedures for the Handling and Processing of Blood Specimens*. Approved Standard H18-A2. Villanova, PA, 1999.

3 Narayanan S. The preanalytic phase: an important component of laboratory medicine. *Am J Clin Pathol*. 2000;113:429-452.

4 Dasgupta A, Dean, R, Saldana S, et al. Absorption of therapeutic drugs by barrier gels in serum separator blood collection tubes. *Clin Chem*. 1993;101(4):456-461.

5 Kiechle F Q&A. *CAP Today*. December 1998.

6 Koepke J. PTT plasma separation. *Tips on Specimen Collection 3*. MLO 1999(suppl):16-17.

7 National Committee for Clinical Laboratory Standards. *Transport and Processing of Blood Specimens for Coagulation Testing and General Performance of Coagulation Assays*. Approved Standard H21-A3. Villanova, PA, 1999.

Chapter 7

Managing Exposures to Bloodborne Pathogens

> *Authors' Note: This chapter will attempt to summarize the current body of knowledge that exists on the appropriate treatment and prophylaxis of accidental needlesticks and other exposures. However, it is noted that as science continues to discover new treatments and test the validity of existing policies in the treatment of accidental needlesticks, new or modified approaches may supersede the information available at the time this information is published. Healthcare professionals should, therefore, be diligent in pursuing and applying current strategies on the care and treatment of accidental needlestick injuries.*

A primary goal of this chapter is to address the decision-making process necessary to:

• Provide the exposed nurse with the best course of action designed to prevent disease transmission, and
• Prevent the administration of treatment and medications that are not clearly justified.

Sustaining an accidental needlestick from a contaminated sharp is a terrifying experience that affects at least 800,000 healthcare workers in the United States every year.[1] Whether the source of the exposure can be traced to the patient on whom the needle was used or not, healthcare professionals face agonizing decisions on the treatment and prophylaxis; often, there is no single best course of action. Because there are so many variables that determine the appropriate and necessary response to an accidental needlestick, cut, or splash, every healthcare professional must be aware of the treatment options as dictated by the variables unique to him/her and be prepared to react accordingly. Likewise, nurse managers must be aware of the treatment options that apply to each individual under a variety of circumstances and work to ensure that their staff is prepared to act.

In hospitals and long-term care facilities, the burden of preparedness clearly falls on nurse managers, occupational health nurses, and other administrators to accommodate contingencies that can be reasonably anticipated. However, healthcare professionals who work in physicians' offices, public health departments, home health agencies, and other capacities without immediate access to an occupational health nurse must be aware of the decisions they will have to make in the event of an accidental exposure and be prepared to act. By preparing in advance under calm circumstances, healthcare professionals avoid the anxiety of making decisions while coping with the emotional trauma inherent in an exposure. A trial run may also reveal lapses in a facility's exposure prevention plan and give managers time to close gaps in the established protocol before the victim of an accidental needlestick is further victimized by an inadequate exposure plan.

On May 15, 1998, the *Morbidity and Mortality Weekly Report* published updated CDC guidelines for management of the healthcare professional exposed to HIV.[2] This document, which provides a well-defined process for evaluating exposures and recommending postexposure prophylaxis, forms the framework for exposure management and, therefore, this chapter.

> Nursing personnel should be diligent in remaining current in regards to new and evolving treatment strategies to prevent disease transmission.

Because exposures associated with phlebotomy are not limited to accidental needlesticks, this chapter will also address those exposures that can occur to nonintact skin and mucous membranes during blood collection, handling, and transportation procedures. Finally, it is this chapter's intent to stress the importance to all healthcare workers of taking personal responsibility for knowing what steps they will have to take in the event of an exposure. Readers should apply information presented here and from other sources to their own unique circumstances and be on the alert in their own workplace for unsafe practices, inadequate policies and hazardous equipment.

PRE-EXPOSURE MANAGEMENT

Understanding Bloodborne Pathogens

Occupational exposure to an infectious disease generally implies an *exposure to the blood or body fluids of a patient who presents a risk of transmitting hepatitis B, C, and the Human Immunodeficiency Virus (HIV)*. These viruses are the most potentially infectious and, if acquired, pose the greatest risk to the exposed healthcare professional. The potential to acquire each of these diseases must be considered separately yet concurrently when determining the appropriate response to an exposure. The risks of transmission surrounding each exposure are a function of factors unique to the circumstances and the individuals involved. Therefore, a complex decision-making schematic is necessary to ensure that the treatment given to those exposed takes into consideration all of the circumstances surrounding their exposure and reflects the current scientific consensus. Any exposure protocol that does not take into consideration the specifics of the injury subjects the healthcare professional to unnecessary procedures, treatment, and risks. The most effective exposure control plan is one that puts current knowledge on disease transmission to use and constructs highly specific actions based on individualized circumstances. These are the plans that best protect a workforce from acquiring an infection and from the panic that can often ensue.

In 1991, the Occupational Safety and Health Administration's (OSHA) Bloodborne Pathogen Standard included in its list of body fluids representing a risk to healthcare workers:[3]

> The most effective exposure control plan is one that puts current knowledge on disease transmission to use and constructs highly specific actions based on individualized circumstances.

- ➢ Blood
- ➢ Semen
- ➢ Vaginal secretions
- ➢ Cerebrospinal fluid
- ➢ Synovial fluid
- ➢ Pleural fluid
- ➢ Pericardial fluid
- ➢ Peritoneal fluid
- ➢ Amniotic fluid
- ➢ Saliva in dental procedures
- ➢ Any body fluid that is visibly contaminated with blood
- ➢ All body fluids in situations where it is difficult or impossible to differentiate among those body fluids.

Accidental needlesticks are a common occupational exposure when performing phlebotomy, but not the only one. Healthcare professionals responsible for centrifuging, processing and/or transferring the serum or plasma to transfer tubes can be vulnerable to splashes into the eye, mucous membranes, or nonintact skin. Personal protection devices in the form of face shields, splash guards, and protective eyewear are available and provide essential protection to healthcare professionals. Even though it is essential that nursing personnel understand the methods of transmission, exposure prevention strategies, and workplace practices that put them at risk, preparing for the accidental exposures that inevitably happen is the next line of defense.

Pre-Exposure Immunizations

In the 1980s, the advent of immunization programs against the hepatitis B virus (HBV) reduced the rate of occupationally acquired hepatitis by 90 percent. OSHA's Bloodborne Pathogen Standard now requires facilities to offer immunizations to its workforce as a preventive measure.[3] The immunization consists of a series of 3 injections administered over 6 months. From 30 to 60 days after the final injection, the healthcare professional should be tested for antibody production. If antibodies are not present in numbers sufficient to indicate immunity, the series should be repeated. If antibodies are still not present after the second series, testing of the healthcare professional should be evaluated to determine if he/she is a chronic carrier of the virus.[4] If it is confirmed that the healthcare professional is a chronic carrier, he/she should be counseled in-depth about the risks of transmitting the virus during patient care and about appropriate prevention strategies. Nurse managers should modify work responsibilities of the chronic carrier to minimize patient risk.

> Immunizations against hepatitis B are to be made available to all healthcare workers free of charge. However, there is no vaccine against hepatitis C or HIV.

If testing reveals that a chronic carrier state does not exist, the person can be considered a *nonconverter*, meaning simply that his/her body will not produce antibodies to the virus and immunity is unattainable. For these individuals, prevention of exposure to HBV becomes paramount.

Unfortunately, there are currently no preventive vaccines recommended for the hepatitis C virus (HCV) or HIV.[4] HCV is transmitted by blood and body fluids and is the etiologic agent in most cases of parenterally transmitted non-A, non-B hepatitis in the United States. It has been estimated that 18 to 60 healthcare workers will acquire HIV from an occupational exposure each year.[5,6] For both of these diseases, the best protection involves the use of personal protective equipment when processing blood and body fluids and caution when handling needles and body fluids.

Studies of healthcare professionals have estimated that the average risk for HIV transmission after a percutaneous exposure to HIV-infected blood is approximately 0.3%.[5,6] Occupational transmission of HIV from patients to healthcare professionals may occur through nonintact skin such as cuts, abrasions, and punctures (percutaneous), or, less frequently, through mucous membranes (mucocutaneous).

Here are a few points to remember about exposure to blood-borne pathogens:

> Following even the most severe exposures, infection with a bloodborne pathogen is not automatic.
> Prevention strategies, such as process evaluation and analysis of facility-specific injuries, are an important component of a safety program for healthcare personnel.
> All facilities presenting an ongoing risk of exposure to their employees should have an occupational health department representative or an alternative available 24 hours a day, every day.

POST-EXPOSURE MANAGEMENT

An exposure to blood or other potentially infectious material should be considered a medical emergency. Because antiretrovirals are associated with serious and debilitating side effects, the decision to administer them after low-risk exposures is difficult. Immediate access to an employee health provider to evaluate the severity and risk factors of an exposure and manage an appropriate response is the cornerstone of an effective exposure management program. This mechanism requires access to the process around the clock, year-round.

In some situations, preventive medications should be administered immediately, ideally within 2 hours of the exposure. In an effective management plan, actions that should be taken after an exposure should include:

> Care of the exposure site (wound or mucous membrane)
> Evaluation of the exposure to determine risk, source testing, and the healthcare professional's candidacy for postexposure prophylactic medication
> Arrangements for follow-up care and counseling for the healthcare professional
> Testing and counseling for the source patient.

A highly choreographed sequence of events should take place after an exposure to assess risk factors and, if necessary, administer prophylactic medication.

Care of the Exposure Site

Immediately upon injury, the site should be thoroughly washed, disinfected, and assessed by a clinician. The care provided to the site depends on the nature of the exposure. Percutaneous injuries (those occurring through accidental needlesticks or by exposure of body fluids to broken skin) are treated differently than mucocutaneous exposure (those resulting from the splashing of body fluids into the mucous membranes of the eyes, nose, or mouth).

Accidental exposure to the tissue either by a puncture with a contaminated needle, a cut by broken glass contaminated with body fluids, demands immediate attention. These exposures are associated with the highest risk of actually acquiring HIV, HBV, and HCV infection (seroconversion) if those viruses are present in the blood or fluid. Potentially infectious body fluids coming into contact with nonintact skin can pose a lesser risk but should be treated with equal urgency. Immediate wound care includes the following:

> Immediately following an exposure, any necessary wound care should be performed and an exposure evaluation should be conducted.

For cuts and needlesticks	For mucous membrane exposures:
➤ Briefly induce bleeding from the wound, if possible ➤ Wash for 10 minutes with an agent known to have activity against HIV (antimicrobial soaps, 10% iodine solution or chlorine-based agents; do not use undiluted bleach or other caustic agents) ➤ Inspect the wound for foreign material and remove.	➤ Irrigate with tap water, sterile saline, or sterile water for 10 to 15 minutes ➤ Exposures involving the eye should include gentle, continuous, and thorough irrigation as from an eyewash station.

Exposure Evaluation

The time just after an injury is a time of intense anxiety and panic for the injured. Unfortunately, in too many facilities it is also a time of anxiety and panic for the individual responsible for implementing the facility's postexposure protocol. Just as it is important to know when testing and treatment is necessary, it is critical to know when it is not.

In determining the appropriate response to an accidental needlestick or exposure to a mucous membrane or nonintact skin, the potential for the injured healthcare worker to acquire each disease must be considered separately yet concurrently. Each response will be a function of a multitude of variables surrounding the exposure and the exposed healthcare worker. It is important to realize that *not all exposures put the healthcare worker at risk of acquiring a bloodborne pathogen.* For example, if healthcare professionals stick themselves with needle used after an unsuccessful venipuncture, they may not necessarily require any attention other than immediate wound care.

In order to make an exposure determination, it is crucial to establish whether or not an *exchange of blood* could have occurred. Some factors to consider include:

> The severity of the exposure
> The route of entry
> The amount of blood involved in the exposure
> The epidemiological likelihood that the healthcare professional was exposed to HBV, HCV or HIV.

> Determining whether an exchange of blood occurred during an exposure is a critical element in determining the appropriate response.

Studies have shown that the risk of acquiring a bloodborne pathogen from needles used in IM injections is significantly less than from needles used in blood collection.[2] Therefore, it should not be assumed that the treatment for an accidental needlestick from a needle that had not yet punctured a vein is the same as for that from a needle that had accessed a vein. Healthcare professionals sustaining injuries can provide the crucial information necessary to assess the severity of the exposure. But someone has to ask the right questions. The most appropriate healthcare professionals to conduct evaluations are the infection control or occupational health nurse and a trained infectious diseases physician.

Case Study
In Michigan, a nurse had accidentally stuck herself with a needle used in an IM injection. It was determined that she should have her blood collected for baseline studies. During the puncture, she was injured by poor technique and suffered a permanent nerve injury so disabling that she was unable to resume her acute care nursing responsibilities.
Commentary: The tragedy in this case is that the baseline lab work may not have been necessary. Unless the needle used on the patient came in direct contact with the patient's blood and resulted in an injury where a blood-to-blood exchange occurred, needles used in an intramuscular (IM) injection do not generally constitute the degree of exposure that necessitates testing or prophylaxis.

Figure 7.1: CDC Algorithm* for determining the need for HIV postexposure prophylaxis (PEP) after an occupational exposure[2]. **Step 1**: Determine the Exposure Control Code (EC) on this page. **Step 2**: Determine the HIV Status Code (HIV SC) on next page. **Step 3**: Determine the PEP Recommendation on next page.

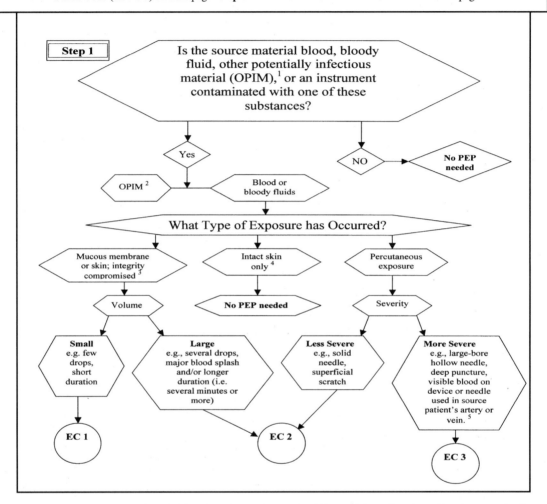

*This algorithm is intended to guide initial decisions about PEP and should be used in conjunction with other sources of information.

1. Semen or vaginal secretions; cerebrospinal, synovial, pleural, peritoneal, pericardial, or amniotic fluids; or tissue.
2. Exposures to OPIM must be evaluated on a case-by-case basis. In general, these body substances are considered a low risk for transmission in healthcare settings. Any unprotected contact to concentrated HIV in a research laboratory or production facility is considered an occupational exposure that requires clinical evaluation to determine the need for PEP.
3. Skin integrity is considered compromised if there is evidence of chapped skin, dermatitis, abrasion, or open wound.
4. Contact with intact skin is not normally considered a risk for HIV transmission. However, if the exposure was to blood, and the circumstance suggests a higher volume exposure (e.g., an extensive area of the skin was exposed or there was prolonged contact with blood), the risk for HIV transmission should be considered.
5. The combination of these severity factors (eg, large-bore hollow needle <u>and</u> deep puncture) contribute to an elevated risk for transmission if the source person is HIV positive.

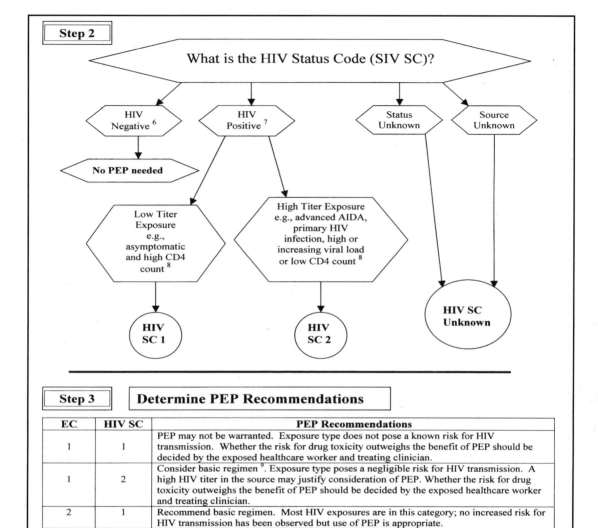

Step 2

What is the HIV Status Code (SIV SC)?

HIV Negative [6]

HIV Positive [7]

Status Unknown

Source Unknown

No PEP needed

Low Titer Exposure e.g., asymptomatic and high CD4 count [8]

High Titer Exposure e.g., advanced AIDA, primary HIV infection, high or increasing viral load or low CD4 count [8]

HIV SC 1

HIV SC 2

HIV SC Unknown

Step 3 | **Determine PEP Recommendations**

EC	HIV SC	PEP Recommendations
1	1	PEP may not be warranted. Exposure type does not pose a known risk for HIV transmission. Whether the risk for drug toxicity outweighs the benefit of PEP should be decided by the exposed healthcare worker and treating clinician.
1	2	Consider basic regimen [9]. Exposure type poses a negligible risk for HIV transmission. A high HIV titer in the source may justify consideration of PEP. Whether the risk for drug toxicity outweighs the benefit of PEP should be decided by the exposed healthcare worker and treating clinician.
2	1	Recommend basic regimen. Most HIV exposures are in this category; no increased risk for HIV transmission has been observed but use of PEP is appropriate.
2	2	Recommend expanded regimen.[10] Exposure type represents an increased HIV transmission risk.
3	1 or 2	Recommend expanded regimen. Exposure type represents an increased HIV transmission risk.
Unknown	Unknown	If the source or, in the case of an unknown source, the setting where the exposure occurred suggests a possible risk for HIV exposure and the EC is 2 or 3, consider PEP basic regimen.

6. A source is considered negative for HIV infection if there is laboratory documentation of a negative HIV antibody test, HIV polymerase chain reaction (PCR) or HIV p24 antigen test result from a specimen collected at or near the time of exposure and there is no clinical evidence of recent retroviral-like illness.

7. A source is considered infected with HIV (HIV positive) if there has been a positive laboratory result for HIV antibody, HIV PCR, or HIV p24 antigen or physician-diagnosed AIDS.

8. Examples are used as surrogates to estimate the HIV titer in an exposure source for purposes of considering PEP regimens and do not reflect all clinical situations that may be observed. Although a high HIV titer (HIV SC2) in an exposure source has been associated with an increased risk for transmission, the possibility of transmission from a source with a low HIV titer also must be considered.

9. Basic regimen is four weeks of zidovudine, 600 mg per day in two or three divided doses, and lamivudine, 150 mg twice daily.

10. Expanded regimen is the basic regimen plus either indinavir, 800 mg every 8 hours, or nelfinavir, 750 mg three times a day.

Once it has been determined that the accident has put the healthcare professional at risk, a systematic approach to treatment is best conducted by considering the risk of acquiring each infection separately.

Post-Exposure Prophylaxis

Hepatitis B

It has been estimated that the risk of becoming infected with hepatitis B from an accidental needlestick is 30 %.[1,5,7] In determining individual risk, the healthcare professional's immune status must be determined. If records or knowledge exists that the healthcare professional has been successfully immunized, transmission is unlikely. Retesting is not necessary and no further treatment is needed under current recommendations.

If the exposed person has not been immunized or if the immune status is not known, the source patient should be tested for the presence of the hepatitis B surface antigen (HBsAg). If the patient tests positive, the exposed healthcare professional should receive hepatitis B Immune Globulin (HBIG) IM at a dose of 0.06 mL/kg body weight ideally within 48 hours of the exposure, but no later than 7 days. A second dose may be indicated in 30 days. This immunization, however, is only effective on 70 to 85 % of those to whom it is administered.[8] In addition, the hepatitis B vaccine should be initiated at this time if the healthcare professional has not yet received the series.

If the patient tests negative for the HBsAb, no prophylaxis is generally indicated. Although it is conceivable the patient could be in the early, undetectable stages of an infection, the exposure is nevertheless considered low-risk and no treatment is indicated. If the individual is currently undergoing the series of hepatitis B immunizations at the time of the exposure, consideration may be given to baseline testing to determine if the immunizations have been successful. This may prevent the unnecessary administration of HBIG.

If the source of the exposure is unknown—for example, from a needle protruding from a sharps container holding many contaminated needles—the exposure must generally be treated as if it were from a patient who has the transmissible hepatitis B virus.

In summary, postexposure hepatitis B prophylaxis is dependent upon the healthcare professional's immune status.

> Establishing the hepatitis B immunization status of the exposed healthcare worker will determine if prophylactic treatment is necessary.

Hepatitis C

There are no effective means to prevent the exposed healthcare professional from acquiring hepatitis C from a patient who harbors the virus. Transmission, however, is not a certainty. Depending on the amount of blood the healthcare professional was exposed to and the concentration of the virus in the patient's blood, the exposure may not be of sufficient volume and/or concentration to be transmitted. The risk of becoming infected with hepatitis C from an accidental needlestick is reported to be 2 to 10 %.[1,5,7]

In the event that an exposure to blood has occurred, the source patient should be tested for the presence of the hepatitis C antibody (anti-HCV). If the patient tests positive, the healthcare worker should be tested at the time of the exposure for a baseline anti-HCV (to determine a preexisting infection) and again after 6 months to determine if hepatitis has been acquired from the event. If the healthcare professional again tests negative after 6 months, it is unlikely the individual will acquire the infection from that exposure.

Of course, if the patient tests negative, the probability of the healthcare professional contracting the disease is greatly diminished. However, this is not a certainty, either. Since some patients may be infected with the virus in quantities too minute to measure at the time of exposure, the potential still exists that the healthcare professional may acquire the virus, albeit that probability is very low. If the source of the exposure is not known, the protocol is the same.

> There is currently no recommended antiviral prophylaxis against hepatitis C.

HIV

Of greatest concern is the transmission of HIV from an accidental needlestick. Ironically, it also poses the least likelihood of transmission of the viruses discussed (0.3 %).[1,5,7] However, because it is more devastating to acquire than either hepatitis B or C, aggressive measures must be considered immediately after a blood exposure has occurred—ideally within hours of the event.[2] Because of the emotional impact that exposure to this virus presents, healthcare professionals must become aware, *before* an exposure occurs, of the appropriate actions they will have to take. Familiarity with the process will help assure that the proper steps are taken within the recommended time frame.

A number of variables exist that determine the actions those exposed should take. Being aware of the variables that apply greatly simplifies the process. Nursing personnel are encouraged, therefore, to project themselves into their facility's exposure control plan pre-

Summary of Exposure Protocol
for exposures that have been determined to put the healthcare worker at an increased risk of bloodborne transmission.

(See Figure 7.1 on pages 116-117 for the CDC exposure evaluation algorithm.)

Hepatitis B

If the healthcare professional has been previously immunized with the hepatitis B vaccine and the immunization has been proven to be successful, prophylactic treatment and source testing is not indicated. Transmission is unlikely to occur.

If the healthcare professional has not been immunized or the success of immunization cannot be determined, the source patient (if known) should be tested for the presence of the hepatitis B antigen (HBsAg). If the patient tests positive, the healthcare professional should receive HBIG at a dose of 0.06 mL/kg body weight IM within 48 hours (preferably, but no longer than within 7 days) of the exposure and repeated in 30 days. The series of hepatitis B immunizations should be initiated. If the patient tests negative, no treatment for the prevention of HBV transmission is indicated.

Healthcare professionals currently undergoing the immunization series should be tested for their immune status (HBsAb) and treated accordingly.

If the source of the exposure cannot be identified and the healthcare professional tests negative (non-immune) or the immune status cannot be determined, the exposed employee should receive HBIG as soon as possible and again in 30 days with consideration given to additional Hepatitis B immunizations.

Hepatitis C

Test the patient source (if known) for the hepatitis C antibody (anti-HCV). If positive, monitor the exposed healthcare worker for symptoms of hepatitis.

Test the exposed individual for baseline anti-HCV at the time of the exposure and again after six months. Monitor for symptoms of hepatitis.

HIV

Due to the complexity of the protocol for reacting to a potential HIV exposure, refer to the CDC Exposure Prevention Algorithm on pages 116-117.

emptively to assure that the plan itself is intact and that the steps they may eventually have to take will be familiar.

When it has been determined that the source should be tested for HIV (see Figure 7.1), the blood for HIV testing should be collected in a small red top tube and immediately transported to the laboratory. (Blood obtained can also be used to test for HBV and HCV as needed. See respective sections.) Currently, rapid HIV tests are available that provide results within minutes. Note that some states require the patient to give his/her "informed consent" before the test can be performed. However, laws outlining the requirements for obtaining informed consent from the source patient vary from state to state. Therefore, each facility's policies must reflect the laws in its state. If consent is required, it is preferred that an individual other than the one experiencing the exposure obtain it. If informed consent cannot be obtained, the patient's physician should be notified and requested to facilitate testing. Occasionally, the healthcare facility's legal counsel may need to address problems obtaining consent in coordination with the executive staff and the facility's risk manager. Because this step may delay appropriate treatment, preplanning for potential obstacles is essential to a well-designed exposure control plan.

> In the event of exposure to HIV positive blood, the facility's PEP should be administered within hours of the exposure to qualified candidates.

In the event of an exposure to HIV-positive blood, the facility's postexposure plan should be implemented. A facility's plan must be unique to their own circumstances and constitutes that facility's preventive (or combination of preventives) initiated and followed in the event of an exposure to prevent disease transmission. The pharmacological preventative that a facility adopts for use after a qualifying exposure is referred to as the facility's Postexposure Prophylaxis, or PEP. For HIV, PEP usually includes a combination of antiretroviral agents, most commonly ziduvodine (ZDV), lamivudine (3TC), and a protease inhibitor (PI). This therapy is aggressive, lengthy, and subject those who receive it to serious and potentially debilitating side effects. Therefore, candidacy must be thoroughly established before administration of the PEP, weighing heavily the variables that determine the likelihood of exposure.

Current research suggests that a facility's PEP for HIV should be administered to qualified candidates within hours of the exposure in order to best protect the victim from acquiring the virus.[2] The same study has shown that PEP may not be effective when started later than 24 to 36 hours after exposure. Because of this urgency, an exposure control plan must be so well-established that it is able to evaluate candidacy and administer the facility's PEP on short notice and around the clock, 365 days a year. A facility with an exposure control plan unable to meet this objective fails to meet the basic intent of the plan and, therefore, fails to protect its workforce.

Although each facility must ultimately establish its own criteria for PEP administration based on established guidelines such as the CDC algorithm (see pages 116-117), some general considerations apply:

> The healthcare professional must have been exposed to blood from a known HIV-positive patient or to body fluid containing visible blood from a known HIV-positive patient,

OR

> The healthcare professional must have been exposed to blood or body fluid containing visible blood from an individual who is at a high risk of being infected with HIV, but whose status is unknown at the time of exposure,

OR

> The healthcare professional has been exposed to a source of undetermined origin.

> The consequence of action versus inaction must be weighed carefully in the event the source patient is unknown.

If the source is unknown, additional factors to consider include the prevalence of HIV in the community and patient population. Unless the patient's HIV status can be determined within hours of the exposure, healthcare professionals should be prepared to make a decision on whether or not to receive the facility's PEP as a preventive measure. Should they decide to begin the facility's PEP therapy and the patient later tests negative, the PEP can be discontinued. Should they decide not to begin PEP therapy and the patient later tests positive, they may have compromised their defense against acquiring the virus. Because of the side effects of the current PEP therapies, however, those exposed to blood of undetermined risk must weigh the consequences of action and inaction carefully and make a personal decision whether or not to receive the facility's PEP.

Follow-up Care and Counseling

For HBV, serial testing for HBsAg should be done at the time of exposure and again after 6 months if the healthcare professional is nonimmune after attempted immunization or has never been immunized, and

> The source is antigen-positive for HBV,

OR

> The source is unknown.

Interim testing may be performed if the healthcare professional experiences symptoms consistent with acute retroviral syndrome or hepatitis regardless of the interval since exposure. (See Table VII: "Symptoms of Acute Retroviral Syndrome.")

For HCV, no postexposure immunization is available. However, testing should be done on the exposed healthcare professional at the time of the exposure and after 6 months if one of the following conditions exist:

> ➤ The source is positive for anti-HCV,
>   OR
> ➤ If the source is unknown.

Interim testing may be performed if the individual experiences symptoms consistent with acute retroviral syndrome or hepatitis regardless of the interval since exposure (see Table VII.)

For HIV, antibody testing should be performed at the time of the exposure (baseline), then 6 weeks, 12 weeks, and 6 months after the exposure if one of the following conditions exists:

> ➤ The source is positive for HIV,
>   OR
> ➤ If the source is unknown.

Interim testing may be performed if the healthcare professional experiences symptoms consistent with acute retroviral syndrome or hepatitis regardless of the interval since exposure (see Table VII). Antiretrovirals should be administered as soon as possible after a qualifying exposure and continued for four weeks until/unless the exposure has been proven to be negligible.

Facilities should be prepared to counsel healthcare personnel that are exposed to potentially infectious blood so that informed, level-headed decisions can be made on an appropriate response to an exposure. The injured healthcare professional may be incapable of making rational decisions in the critical time following an exposure and can find comfort in being counseled by clinicians experienced in dealing with occupational exposures and knowledgeable of the facility's exposure control plan. The injured not only requires counseling on the immediate therapy options, but also needs to be informed of follow-up testing, the possibility of transmitting any viruses acquired from the exposure to family, patients, and other contacts, ways to prevent such secondary transmissions, the implications of current or

> After an exposure, healthcare workers should be counseled by clinicians experienced in dealing with occupational exposures and familiar with the facility's exposure control plan.

future pregnancies, etc. The need for counseling is urgent and significant. Facilities should make such services available 24-hours a day.

The CDC recommends that healthcare professionals with occupational exposure should receive follow-up counseling, appropriate testing, and medical evaluation regardless of whether or not the facility's PEP was administered. Counseling should include information regarding:

> Precautions to prevent disease transmission at work and home
> Symptoms of virus transmission
> Side effects of the facility's prescribed PEP
> Recommended follow-up testing.

Post-exposure counseling is a critical component of an exposure control plan to prevent the spread of potentially acquired pathogens.

Because of the potential to acquire a viral infection and harbor a persistent viremia, the healthcare professional who acquires the hepatitis B, hepatitis C, or HIV virus remains potentially infectious to others. Those exposed should be advised to use measures to prevent secondary transmission until it has been established that they have not acquired a transmissible virus. These measures include the following:

> Sexual abstinence or use of condoms
> Defer pregnancy
> Refrain from donating blood, plasma, organs, tissue, or semen
> Discontinue breast-feeding, especially following high-risk exposures
> Strict adherence to universal precautions
> Promptly reporting incidences in which healthcare professionals have put patients at risk through exposure to their blood or other potentially infectious fluids.

Nursing personnel who choose to take the prescribed PEP must work closely with their occupational health professional for advice on food and drug interactions, side effects, adherence to time and dosage regimens, and the body's need for increased fluid intake. Reactions to the medications that require immediate attention include back or abdominal pain, pain on urination, blood in urine, or symptoms of hyperglycemia. The healthcare professional who is pregnant and taking the facility's PEP requires special attention by the occupa-

---

Table VII: Symptoms of Acute Retroviral Syndrome

Exposed healthcare workers should also be counseled regarding the importance of seeking medical evaluation for any acute illness that occurs during the follow-up period characterized by:

> ➤ Fever
> ➤ Rash
> ➤ Myalgia
> ➤ Fatigue
> ➤ Malaise
> ➤ Lymphadenopathy

---

tional health specialist since both mother and baby may be directly affected.

Finally, it is important for the exposed individual to adhere to the schedule for follow-up blood work including, but not limited to, CBCs and liver function studies. These tests may be ordered weekly and depend upon the medication(s) included in the PEP, preexisting medical history of the exposed healthcare professional, and other factors.

Emotional support is an important necessity during this 6 month period, especially in the event of a high-risk exposure. All counseling and follow-up care should be done in an environment that maintains confidentiality and allows for sufficient time to answer questions and address concerns.

> Emotional support and follow-up blood tests are important to complete implementation of an exposure control plan.

Testing and Counseling for the Source Patient

If it has been determined that a high-risk exposure has occurred (see Figure 7.1, pages 116-117), testing of the source (if known) must include HCV and HIV using CDC's Hospital Infection Control Practices Advisory Committee recommendations.[4] HBV testing is only necessary if the healthcare worker's immunity to HBV cannot be established. The source of the exposure requires counseling with regard to the baseline test results, which include HIV, HCV, and, perhaps, HBV. It is essential that test results be communicated by a clinician skilled in counseling, especially if results indicate an infection with one of the viruses. Privacy and an atmosphere that minimizes distractions are necessary. A well-established and working protocol for this counseling should be part of the overall exposure management plan.

ESTABLISHING AN EXPOSURE CONTROL PLAN

Elements of a Comprehensive and Functional Exposure Control Plan

Effective exposure control plans consist of rapid response, multi-contingency, and highly defined implementation procedures.

To be comprehensive and functional, an exposure control plan must address a broad range of contingencies and obstacles to successful implementation. In addition, it must be universally applied regardless of the personnel on duty. Designers and administrators of the exposure control plan should use the following checklist to assess the overall utility of their facility's plan and are advised to address the deficiencies before the need arises.

> The plan should accommodate on-site as well as off-site work-related injuries.

> The plan should ensure that mechanisms are in place to accomplish rapid and immediate HIV testing. This includes test ordering, specimen collection, specimen transportation, billing, and result reporting.

> The plan should clearly define the steps that injured healthcare personnel should take to ensure the best and most appropriate treatment of their exposure.

> The plan should include the protocol necessary to collect and test the patient's blood for bloodborne pathogens. This should include the location of consent forms and the circumstances under which consent is unnecessary. It should also define who should collect the blood, how the blood should be collected, and where the blood should be sent for testing.

> The plan should reflect the current consensus on preventive therapies when establishing its PEP and be reviewed and revised on a regular basis.

> The plan should identify the criteria for administration of the PEP and detail those conditions in which PEP is not indicated.

➢ The plan should guarantee that the PEP is not only available, but also accessible, 24 hours a day, seven days a week, 365 days a year.

➢ The plan should arrange for the PEP prescriptions to be written by physicians and filled at locations that preserve the healthcare professional's confidentiality if it becomes an issue.

➢ The plan should guarantee that HBIG is available for administration within 48 hours after any exposure.

➢ The plan should not require costly medications to be paid for by the healthcare worker regardless of reimbursement.

➢ The plan should have a mechanism in place so that an occupational health nurse is immediately available to implement the plan, resolve problems, and counsel the injured.

> Nursing personnel share ownership in their facility's exposure control plan and should alert plan administrators of lapses as they become evident.

All of these considerations are important to ensure that nursing personnel who are exposed to bloodborne pathogens receive the most timely, confidential, and effective care and treatment to prevent disease transmission. For administrators, the staff must be continually assured that there exists an intense and conscientious concern for their well-being. Such concern is directly proportional to the scope and complexity of the facility's exposure control plan.

Nursing personnel can and should share ownership in an exposure control plan by being alert for lapses in safety practices and the exposure control plan before an injury occurs. They must also be responsible for adherence to the plan. Their willingness to share information on safety devices as they become available is equally critical. Without active participation, even the most comprehensive exposure control plan is destined to fail.

Assessing Effectiveness

Healthcare facilities have a legal and moral obligation to their employees to provide a safe working environment that minimizes risk of injuries that can be reasonably anticipated during the performance of their duties. Likewise, employers have an obligation to respond promptly, effectively, and completely to injuries sustained and illnesses acquired on the job. When that injury or illness is a result of an exposure to potentially infectious blood or body fluids, nothing demonstrates the fulfillment of this obligation like a comprehensive, functional exposure control plan.

Developing and implementing a comprehensive and functional plan is an enormous undertaking that demands a high level of commitment and a fierce attention to detail. However, not all comprehensive plans are fully functional and not all functional plans are comprehensive. It is imperative, therefore, that nursing personnel who collect and/or process blood specimens research their employer's plan to ensure that elements are intact that will provide them with the best protection against acquiring a bloodborne pathogen.

To test the functionality of an existing exposure control plan, healthcare professionals should walk through the steps they would take if they became exposed to blood through an accidental needlestick or through nonintact skin or mucous membrane contact, regardless of the day or time. The following is a list of questions that may be considered when testing a facility's ability to respond to an accidental needlestick or other exposure.

> Whom should I notify when I have an accidental needlestick?
> Where should I go for immediate care?
> Are they prepared to treat me immediately and administer the appropriate PEP within 2 hours of my exposure if necessary?
> Who will administer the PEP if I need it?
> If the PEP is not on hand, is there a mechanism in place for obtaining it immediately 24 hours a day, 365 days a year?
> What forms am I supposed to fill out?
> Will those forms be available when I need them?
> Is there an eyewash station or bottle in the area where I would most likely be exposed?
> Where should I go for baseline lab work?
> What baseline lab work should be drawn and what tubes are required?
> What physician will order the lab work?
> Will I be expected to pay for the lab work?
> Who will pay for the PEP if I need it?
> If I am to be reimbursed for the lab work or PEP, what if I don't have enough money to pay for it up front?
> Can I go to an off-site laboratory to protect my confidentiality?

Every exposure control plan should be tested for its ability to function at all times and under all conceivable circumstances.

➤ If so, how will the laboratory be paid?

➤ If the physician receives the results, how and when will I be notified?

➤ Who else will see my lab results?

➤ Who will determine if I need the PEP?

➤ How do I assess the risk of the exposure?

➤ What tests should be run on the patient?

➤ What tubes should be drawn on a patient for postexposure testing?

➤ Do I need the patient's permission to draw and test for HIV? Hepatitis?

➤ What if the patient refuses to be tested?

➤ Where will the patient's testing be performed?

➤ Does the testing lab have a mechanism in place for testing and reporting postexposure cases within 2 hours?

➤ If testing is done off-site, how does the specimen reach the lab?

➤ Who will pay for the patient's testing?

➤ What is my immune status for hepatitis?

➤ Are contingencies in place if I stick myself on third shift, a weekend, or during a holiday?

➤ Has the plan been tested lately?

➤ What if the emergency department is too busy to attend to my injury and treatment in a timely manner?

➤ I'm pregnant. Should I still take the PEP?

➤ What are the risks of transmitting an acquired virus to my husband? My family?

> The answers to these questions and those on the preceding page will be easily attainable in a facility with an effective exposure control plan.

As you can tell, there is a multitude of details that have to be considered and accommodated in a functional and comprehensive exposure control plan. Not all facilities have the resources to put such a plan in place. As healthcare professionals who may have to rely on their facility's existing plan to protect them with the most up-to-date concepts in postexposure treatment, it is imperative that deficiencies be illuminated and eliminated through a cooperative effort before the plan fails to protect an injured employee. Nursing personnel should evaluate the ability of their facility's exposure control plan to respond to a variety of realistic circumstances and conditions before they are put to the test. Any gaps or inadequacies should be communicated and cooperatively resolved. Healthcare professionals without administrative responsibilities can be instrumental in improving existing mechanisms and should welcome the opportunity to engineer the perfection and implementation of a functional, comprehensive plan.

Exposure Report Management

Nurse administrators and infection control nurses must keep accurate records on exposure events to satisfy regulatory agencies. Recording exposures serves to track trends within a facility and to provide a mechanism by which infection control nurses can be alerted to high risk procedures, departments and personnel. An effective exposure reporting tool allows for simple entry, complies with OSHA regulations, is customizable to the facility's needs, and is searchable according to ward, personnel, injury type, etc. Many exposure reporting systems are available commercially to help facilities implement an effective means to monitor and control exposures. One unique method is the NICSx™ Needlestick Incident Control System (Bio Medical Disposal, Inc., Norcross, Georgia). This tool is a highly developed web-based reporting system that enables users to record and address behaviors that cause exposures, retrieve and print reports, and monitor trends. The system also provides automatic updates of new regulations on a state-specific basis.

References

1 Pallatroni L. Needlesticks: Who pays the price when costs are cut on safety? *MLO*, July 1998;30(7):30-35.
2 Centers for Disease Control and Prevention. Public health service guidelines for the management of healthcare workers exposures to HIV and recommendations for postexposure prophylaxis. *Morb Mortal Wkly Rep.* 1998;47(RR-7):1-37.
3 US Department of Labor, Occupational Health and Safety Administration. Occupational exposure to bloodborne pathogens; final rule. CFR part 1910.1030. *Federal Register.* 1991;56:64004-64182.
4 Centers for Disease Control and Prevention. Immunization of healthcare workers: recommendations of the Advisory Committee on Immunization Practices (AICP) and the Hospital Infection Control Practices Advisory Committee (HICPAC). *MMWR Morb Mortal Wkly Rep.* 1997;46(RR-18):1-42.
5 Holding R. Carlsen W. Watchdogs fail health workers. *San Francisco Chronicle.* April 12, 1998. Available at: http://www.sfgate.com. Accessed June 8, 1998.
6 International Healthcare Worker Safety Center. Risk of infection following a single HIV, HBV, or HCV-contaminated needlestick or sharp instrument injury. http://www.med.virginia.edu. accessed August 2, 2000.
7 Centers for Disease Control and Prevention. Preventing needlestick injuries in health care settings. *NIOSH Alert.* Publication No. 2000-108; November, 1999.
8 Centers for Disease Control and Prevention. Protection against viral hepatitis: recommendations of the Advisory Committee on Immunization Practices (ACIP). *MMWR Morb Mortal Wkly Rep.* 1990;39(RR-2):1-27

Chapter 8

Practices and Products for Exposure Prevention

As we have seen in the previous chapter, exposure to blood and body fluids can have devastating consequences. There are, however, a multitude of preventive practices and products that can significantly reduce every healthcare professional's risk of exposure. As more and more healthcare professionals from a variety of disciplines assume phlebotomy responsibilities, it becomes paramount that protective practices and devices are introduced into the routine of collecting and handling potentially infectious material.

SAFE PRACTICES

Too often those new to phlebotomy adopt a cavalier approach to specimen collection and handling, which invites a false sense of immunity from a life-threatening exposure. Only when healthcare professionals are fully aware of the practices that put them at great risk for the panic and devastation that accompanies all accidental exposures can a healthy respect for safe practices emerge.

Those who draw specimens can be exposed to blood during handling, processing, and transportation of specimens in predictable and unpredictable ways. Implementing safe blood collection and handling and practices and using products designed to minimize exposure can drastically reduce the potential for exposure to blood-borne pathogens.

> Only when nursing professionals are fully aware of the practices that may subject them to the panic and devastation of an accidental exposure can a healthy respect for safe practices emerge.

Some potential means of exposure *after* the specimen is collected include:

> Accidental needlesticks
> Tube breakage during centrifugation
> Tube breakage during transportation
> Splashes when caps are removed
> Spills or splashes while transferring serum or plasma to a transport tube
> Splashes to the eye or nonintact skin during spill clean-up.

Without understanding and implementing universal precautions, collectors are not fully protected against accidental exposure.

Although this lists only a few of the more common modes of accidental exposure, scenarios that can put nursing personnel at risk are unlimited when collecting and handling blood specimens. Minimizing exposure can be accomplished by consistently implementing the following five practices as set forth in the OSHA Bloodborne Pathogen Standard:

> Exercise universal precautions
> Use personal protective equipment
> Follow proper protocol for accidental blood spills
> Handle contaminated needles properly
> Convert from conventional needles to safety needles facility-wide.

Universal Precautions

As mentioned in Chapter 3, universal precautions is a method of infection control in which all human blood and certain body fluids are treated as if known to be infectious for HIV, HBV, and other bloodborne pathogens. (See Box, page 41.)

Use of Personal Protective Equipment
Gloves

It is advisable for healthcare professionals to expand their definition of a successful puncture to include one that is performed without exposing the collector to bloodborne pathogens. This expanded definition does not allow for gloveless venipunctures. Nor does it accommodate the frequent practice of tearing off the tip of the glove to expose the index finger. While this practice may retain the ability to palpate the vein, it also obliterates the protective barrier that the glove and OSHA's Bloodborne Pathogen Standard provide. Although gloves cannot provide protection without decreasing sensitivity and, therefore, the ability to palpate the vein, it is a necessary compromise. Unfortunately, healthcare professionals often circumvent the protection that gloves offer in this way, convinced that doing so will facilitate a successful puncture. Such faulty justification contributes to the annual statistics on occupationally acquired diseases. Any attempts to compromise the protection for the sake of sensitivity should be thwarted. Healthcare personnel should become accustomed to the use of gloves and employ techniques that maintain glove use while minimizing the limitations. This can be accomplished in several ways.

> *The gloves need not be put on until immediately before the puncture.* This allows for ungloved palpation to locate the vein. Locating the vein prior to glove use, though, is not acceptable when the patient is in isolation.

> *Establish the exact location of veins before puncturing.* To eliminate the need to repalpate the intended puncture site after the gloves have been put on to relocate the vein, plot veins in relation to certain skin markers such as freckles, skin creases, or other surface features.

Gloves must be worn when performing phlebotomy. Failure to do so puts healthcare workers at risk of exposure and is in violation of OSHA's Bloodborne Pathogen Standard.

These techniques eliminate the necessity to re-palpate the vein with an *ungloved* finger and preserve the protection that gloves provide.

Repeated use of latex gloves industry-wide has resulted in the sensitization of healthcare professionals to latex. Studies show that between 6 and 17 % of latex glove users develop a latex allergy.[1] This problem has urged a transition in the healthcare industry to the use of vinyl or nonlatex gloves. The loose-fitting nature of vinyl, however, presents further problems for those collecting blood in that it further decreases sensitivity and dexterity. Nitrile gloves offer the form-fitting flexibility of latex without the risk of acquiring a latex allergy.

Protective gowns and face shields

When handling specimens (eg, transporting tubes, removing stoppers from blood tubes, transferring serum or plasma or otherwise accessing specimens), healthcare professionals must protect themselves adequately and according to OSHA's Bloodborne Pathogen Standard to prevent accidental exposure. This involves the use of gloves, a protective gown, and eye protection. Because of the risk of splatter when specimens are uncapped and handled, processing should take place with a barrier between the specimen and the processor. This barrier can exist in the form of protective eyewear or a clear acrylic or plastic shield positioned between the specimen and the processor. Garments must be impermeable and, therefore, composed of fluid repellent material. It is the employer's responsibility to provide and launder impermeable gowns and to replace those in which the integrity of the barrier is compromised. Examples include gowns that are torn or have become permeable.

When handling specimens, health-care professionals must protect themselves adequately to prevent accidental exposure. This involves the use of gloves, a protective gown, and eye protection.

If a specimen has been accessed for separation, the original tube should be sealed with the cap or otherwise covered to keep the specimen from spilling, regardless of whether the tube is to be stored or discarded. The serum or plasma extracted should likewise be capped and stored under proper conditions, according to the test requirements.

Proper Protocol for Blood Spills

Blood spills should be immediately cleaned up with gloves and other necessary personal protective equipment in place to minimize the risk of exposure. For small spills and splashes that do not involve broken glass, flood the area with a solution of 10 % bleach and wipe with absorbent towels. The towels should be discarded into a receptacle for biohazardous waste.

Blood tubes should be centrifuged with their stoppers on and in a centrifuge with a locking lid.

For large spills and/or spills that involve broken glass, flood the spill with 10 % bleach and sprinkle with an absorbent compound. Spill kits such as EZ-Cleans Plus™ (SafeTec, Buffalo, NY) contain gloves, a scoop, disinfectant wipes, a biohazardous waste bag, and an absorbent powder that congeals spills and provide a convenient

---

Safe Centrifuge Use

To protect against exposure during centrifugation, tubes should be capped to prevent aerosols from being emitted. Centrifuges must also have a locking lid that will prevent splatter and aerosols from escaping in the event a tube breaks while the centrifuge is running. The locking lid should prevent opening of the lid while the rotor is in motion. All safety devices on the centrifuge must be in place and activated. Modification of safety features is in violation of OSHA regulations and puts the healthcare professional at risk.

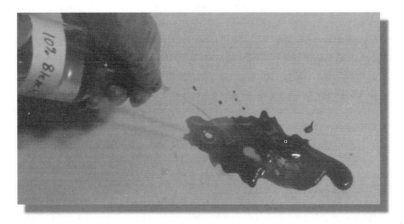

Figure. 8.2: For small spills and splashes that do not involve broken glass, flood the area with a solution of 10 percent bleach and wipe with absorbent towels. The towels should be discarded into a receptacle for biohazardous waste.

Spills involving blood should be decontaminated before wiping. Broken glass should never be picked up by hand.

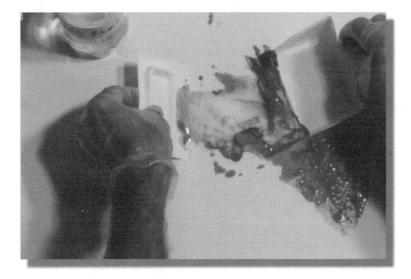

Figure. 8.3: For large spills and/or spills that involve broken glass, flood the spill with 10 percent bleach and sprinkle with an absorbent compound. Collect congealed blood and glass with a scoop and discard into a sharps container.

means to handle blood spills. Sweep the broken glass and blood-soaked absorbent compound into a dustpan and discard into a sharps container. Flood any residual blood remaining on the surface again with the bleach solution and wipe with absorbent towels. Discard towels into a receptacle for biohazardous waste.

If a specimen tube breaks during centrifugation, the lid should remain closed for at least a half-hour to allow for the settling of fine droplets. While wearing appropriate personal protection equipment, the healthcare professional should open the centrifuge carefully and remove the larger pieces of glass with a hemostat or other device. *Never use hands to retrieve broken glass!* Other tubes should be inspected for damage and contamination and cleansed appropriately with a solution of 10 % bleach. The interior of the centrifuge should be similarly decontaminated.[2] The use of puncture-resistant gloves is recommended.

The development of plastic blood collection tubes has dramatically reduced the risk of exposure when blood collection tubes are dropped. Facilities should make every attempt to convert to plastic tubes for the safety of those who collect, process and test specimens as well as for the convenience of their patients who would otherwise have to be re-collected. A full line of plastic tubes is available from Greiner Vacuette North America (Bel Air, Maryland). BD (Franklin Lakes, New Jersey) offers a plastic counterpart for most of their glass collection tubes.

> Since most accidental needlesticks occur with hollow-bore needles, it is critical for those who draw blood specimens, insert IVs and administer injections to employ safe equipment and technique.

Proper Handling of Contaminated Needles

It has been estimated that 1 million healthcare professionals suffer an accidental needlestick every year.[3,4] Nearly half of these—46%—are by nurses.[5] Conventional hollow-bore needles account for 68% of all accidental needlesticks to healthcare workers.[3] A study conducted by the Centers for Disease Control and Prevention shows that the use of safety needles and drawing devices can reduce the frequency of accidental needlesticks by up to 76%.[6]

One-handed Needle Disposal

From the moment the needle is removed from the patient, the healthcare professional must consider it to be lethal. The window of vulnerability to accidental needlesticks is open as soon as the needle is removed from the patient and remains open until it is discarded. If the needle is not immediately discarded, concealed, destroyed, or otherwise rendered incapable of causing a puncture, the healthcare professional is vulnerable to sustaining an injury and contracting a life-threatening illness.

After the blood has been obtained, the needle should be removed from the patient and concealed or deposited into a sharps container *in one fluid motion.* According to OSHA's Bloodborne Pathogen Standard, needles should not be removed before discarding. Unless the entire unit is discarded, concealment by resheathing with the original sheath re-exposes the healthcare professional when the needle is removed and discarded. With the wide variety of products

OSHA's Stance on Needle Recapping and Removal

According to the OSHA Bloodborne Pathogen Standard, contaminated sharps are not to be bent, recapped, or removed unless *both* of the following conditions exist:[8]

➤ Employer can demonstrate that no alternative is feasible or that bending, recapping or removing is required by a specific procedure, and
➤ Bending, recapping, or needle removal must be accomplished through the use of a mechanical device or a one-handed technique.

The Standard further states that contaminated sharps shall be discarded immediately or as soon as feasible in containers that are closable, puncture resistant, leak proof on sides and bottom and labeled or color-coded in accordance with OSHA labeling standards. Containers for contaminated sharps are to be easily accessible to personnel and located as close as is feasible to the immediate area where sharps are used or can be reasonably anticipated to be found. They should remain upright throughout use and not be allowed to overfill.

Although some state, county and municipal facilities are exempt from OSHA regulations, it is prudent for all employers to voluntarily comply.

available to circumvent such resheathing, those responsible for procuring equipment should make every attempt to provide alternatives. OSHA states that if no alternative to recapping is feasible or if needle removal is required by a specific procedure, the conditions that necessitate recapping and/or removal must be documented in the facility's exposure control plan stating the basis for the determination.

Under such circumstances, OSHA allows needle *recapping* only through a one-handed method, eg, the hand holding the sharp is used to scoop up the cap from a flat surface. Needle recapping must be limited to such situations and *should never be performed using the two-handed recapping procedure.* Such a technique was in favor decades ago but has long since become a deadly practice. One-handed resheathing, however, is the least effective means of safely disposing a contaminated needle.

Needle *removal* must be done by a mechanical device or a one-handed technique. Devices and engineering controls that allow for one-handed concealment and disposal of contaminated needles provide the greatest protection against accidental needlesticks.

> If conventional needles must be resheathed, it must be accomplished by a one-handed technique.

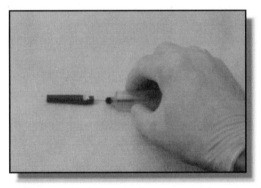

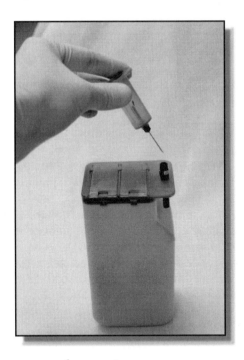

Figure. 8.5: Under certain circumstances, contaminated needles may be recapped using the one-handed scoop method (above) or by using the hole at the top of some sharps containers to accommodate the sheath (left).

"Contaminated needles and other contaminated sharps shall not be bent, recapped, or removed unless the employer can demonstrate that no alternative is feasible or that such action is required by a specific medical or dental procedure."

OSHA Bloodborne Pathogen Standard

Convert to Safety Needles

Federal and state legislation mandates conversion to safety needles.

Since 1988, the US Patent and Trademark Office has issued more than 1000 patents for devices that protect healthcare workers from accidental needlesticks.[7] With the multitude of products on the market designed to protect healthcare workers from occupationally acquired diseases, facilities should thoroughly analyze those devices that offer the best, most cost-effective protection according to their needs and their patient population. *The additional cost of investing in safe blood collection devices is easily justifiable when considering the cost to a facility of treating employees for accidental needlesticks and occupationally acquired diseases.* Federal and state legislation exists mandating employers to use only those devices that protect healthcare professionals from accidental needlesticks. (See "Safety Needle Legislation" box in Chapter 1.)

This explosion in patents for safety devices has brought a multitude of new products designed to minimize healthcare professionals' exposure to contaminated sharps. Because of legislation and the heightened awareness of the risks to the nation's 8.8 million

Needlestick Injury Statistics

The following statistics underscore the importance of protecting the healthcare professional against accidental exposure.

➤ Needlesticks by occupation:[5]
- Nurses: 46%
- Laboratory technicians: 23%
- Doctors: 15%
- Housekeeper/laundry: 5%
- Other: 12%

➤ Chance of becoming infected when stuck with a contaminated needle:[3,4]
- Hepatitis B: 30%
- Hepatitis C: 2% to 10 %
- HIV: 1 in 300

➤ Estimated accidental needlestick injuries sustained by healthcare workers worldwide per year: 1 million.[3,4]
➤ Number of accidental needlesticks that go unreported: up to 92%.[4]
➤ Accidental needlesticks per day: 2400.
➤ Percent of accidental needlesticks caused by hollow-bore needles: 68%.[3]
➤ Healthcare workers projected to be infected with HIV through accidental needlesticks per year: 18 to 60.[9]
➤ Healthcare personnel infected with hepatitis B every year from accidental needlesticks: 1000.[9]
➤ Number of diseases capable of being transmitted through needlesticks: at least 20.[10]
➤ Cost of treating accidental needlestick (testing and prophylaxis): $4000.[3]
➤ Cost of treating HIV-infected employee (from needlestick): $500,000 to $1 million.[11]
➤ Average settlement for occupationally acquired HIV: $2 to $5 million.[4]

Case Study
A healthcare professional just beginning his shift found the sharps container on the phlebotomy tray filled to capacity. Closing the unit required him to press a hinged flap over the top opening and locking it into place. The container was so full that closing the flaps required squeezing the lid with significant force, using both hands. The pressure necessary to lock the lid forced a contaminated sharp through the bottom of the container, piercing his thumb.
Commentary: When needle-disposal units are three quarters full, they should be sealed and discarded according to the facility's protocol for disposal. Units that are allowed to fill beyond this level put healthcare professionals at risk for accidental needlesticks.

healthcare personnel, product development and innovation are accelerating. Those in a position to evaluate and implement safety products should carefully consider current products and aggressively seek information on newly emerging technologies.

The safest needle concealment or disposal products are those that are activated while the needle is still in the vein or those that, once the needle is removed, require one hand to activate. With one hand applying pressure on the puncture site, the device that requires two hands to dispose of or conceal the contaminated sharp incorporates a dangerous delay in its design. For this reason, any device that cannot be activated by one hand immediately after removal of the needle from the vein is inherently disadvantageous.

Although the following is not a comprehensive list of safety products on the market, it lists some of the current designs available to protect the healthcare professional from the risks involved in blood specimen collection.

Safety Products

Products that Facilitate Needle Concealment

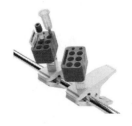

THE MOBILE DRAW STATION™

The Mobile Draw Station (MarketLab, Inc., Kentwood, MI) is a tube caddy that facilitates one-handed resheathing when a sharps container is not within reach at the point of use. A portable tube rack is incorporated into a clip-on device that can be attached to many bedside surfaces, keeping supplies, tubes, and needle sheaths nearby. When in use, the contaminated needle can be immediately sheathed with one hand instead of using the cumbersome one-handed scoop method.

The Mobile Draw Station™ (Photo courtesy of MarketLab, Inc., Kentwood, MI)

POINT-LOK™

Point-Lok (Sims Portex Keene, NH) is a needle concealment device that can facilitate needle concealment when a sharps container is not within reach at the point of use. To use, the thimble-size product is placed within reach prior to the puncture. When the needle is removed from the patient, the tip is pressed into the device, which permanently locks onto the sharp, preventing it from inflicting injury. The single-use item is discarded with the needle into the nearest sharps container.

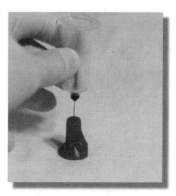

Point-Lok™ (Sims Portex Keene, NH)

Needle Disposal Units

A needle-disposal unit must be on the tray of blood collection supplies or positioned within reach. Units that are positioned away from the patient and require the collector to carry a contaminated sharp any distance from the point of use are ineffective and put the healthcare worker at great risk. *Units must be within reach at the time the needle is removed from the patient.* This is especially true where conventional needles are used.

Because accidental punctures from needles of unidentifiable sources cannot be properly investigated, they must be treated as if contaminated with bloodborne pathogens. Victims of punctures from anonymous sources suffer unnecessary treatment and immeasurable anxiety.

AUTOMATIC NEEDLE DISCONNECT (A.N.D.™)

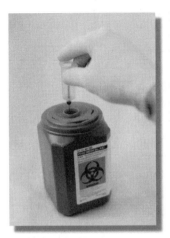

The Automatic Needle Disconnect (A.N.D™.) Post Medical (Atlanta, GA)

The Automatic Needle Disconnect (A.N.D.) (Post Medical, Atlanta, GA) accommodates one-handed needle disposal when drawing blood with a tube holder. With this product, once the needle is removed from the arm it is placed needle-first into a mechanism incorporated into the top of the needle disposal unit. When turned and pressed downward, the needle automatically unthreads and falls from the holder into the sharps container. As an added safety feature, when the unit is full enough to be discarded, the unthreading mechanism locks in the downward position to prevent overfilling. The A.N.D. provides immediate, one-handed needle disposal, an important feature for reducing the frequency of accidental needlesticks. However, since this device is designed only for use with needle holders used in vacuum-assisted draws, needles used during syringe draws must be discarded by other means.

Automatic Needle Releases

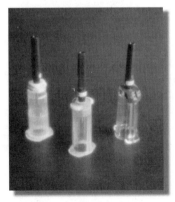

Automatic needle release tube holders l-r: Pronto™ (BD, Franklin Lakes, NJ), AutoDrop™ (Kendall, St Louis, MO), and Drop-it™ (Bio-Plexus, Vernon, CT).

DROP-IT™, PRONTO™, AUTODROP™

Several manufacturers have designed tube holders for vacuum-assisted draws that facilitate one-handed needle disposal. The Drop-it (Bio-Plexus, Vernon, CT), Pronto (BD, Franklin Lakes, NJ), and AutoDrop (Kendall, Mansfield, MA) all incorporate needle release mechanisms activated by the push of a release trigger. When the contaminated needle is removed from the arm, it is held with the needle pointing downward above a sharps container. The mechanism is activated with the push of a finger, releasing the needle so that it falls into the sharps container. Proper use of these devices requires the presence of a sharps container at the point of use.

Needle Destruction Units (NDU)

These devices allow for one-handed needle disposal by disintegrating the needle immediately after use in a process known as pyroelectric oxidation. When removed from the vein, the contaminated needle is quickly placed into the NDU in one fluid motion. The NDU is activated and the needle is reduced to a metallic ash, which falls into a catch bin. Vapors are drawn by a fan through a filter.

Such devices allow for one-handed needle disposal at the point of use, significantly reducing the volume of waste in sharps containers. When used on needles in tube holders, however, the sharp within the holder remains as a potential risk unless the facility discards all holders after use. If used in hospital settings for inpatient collections, NDUs, although portable, may necessitate a cart to transport for convenience. Battery operated, both NDUs listed below can destroy up to 100 needles on a single charge. NDUs are contraindicated in areas where potentially explosive gas (oxygen, etc.) or liquids are being used or stored.

NEEDLYZER™

The Needlyzer (MedPro, Lexington, KY) destroys contaminated needles at permanent drawing stations, at the bedside, or at remote sites. Utilizing electric-eye technology, the device automatically starts when the operator's hand approaches the unit. When the needle is placed between two positively charged electrodes inside the unit, the resultant arc oxidizes the metal at 1,500° Celsius. The process takes less than 1 second, and the unit shuts off after the needle has been completely destroyed to the hub and the syringe or tube holder removed.

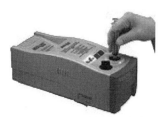

Needlyzer™
(Photo courtesy of MedPro, Lexington, KY)

SHARPX™

Using an electric current, the SharpX (Bio Medical Disposal, Inc., Norcross, GA) disintegrates used sharps with one-handed operation leaving a blunt stub. The unit weighs two pounds and can accommodate 19 to 27 gauge needles. Debris is minimal and is captured in a removable receptacle while vaporized gases are directed through a filtration system. The system is equipped with two visible and one audible low-battery alert signals and recharges completely in 45-90 minutes.

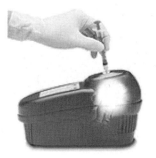

SharpX™
(Photo courtesy of Bio Medical Disposal, Inc., Norcross, GA)

Modified Tube Holders

Traditional tube holders are coming under increased scrutiny because of contamination after one use and because their reuse requires the removal of used needles from them to facilitate reuse. Products in this class consist of single-use tube holders for vacuum-assisted draws.

VANISHPOINT®

The VanishPoint (Retractable Technologies, Inc., Lewisville, TX) is designed to eliminate exposure to the contaminated sharp by being activated while the needle is still within the patient's arm. It does so by incorporating a spring-loaded mechanism into the tube holder for vacuum-assisted draws. To use the device, the holder is threaded with a standard, conventional needle from any manufacturer and the puncture is performed as usual. After the last tube has been filled and removed, the collector places a gauze pad over the site and closes a hinged cap to cover the open end of the holder. When pressed into place, the spring-loaded mechanism is activated and automatically retracts the needle from the patient's vein into the now-sealed tube holder. The collector applies pressure to the puncture site and discards the holder with the encapsulated needle into a sharps container. Because of the instantaneous retraction of the needle from the arm into the protective holder, the healthcare professional is never at risk of an accidental needlestick when the device is used properly.

This device activates while the needle is within the patient's arm, eliminating exposure to the contaminated sharp. Since the holder is larger than conventional holders to accommodate the retractable mechanism, facilities can experience an increase in their volume of biohazardous waste.[12]

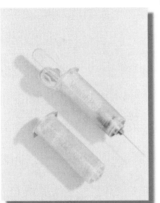

VanishPoint® (Photo courtesy of Retractable Technologies, Inc Lewisville, TX)

VENIPUNCTURE NEEDLE-PRO®

The SIMS Portex Venipuncture Needle-Pro (SIMS Portex, Inc., Keene, NH) is a single-use tube holder that utilizes a hinged shield integrated into the holder. When the needle is withdrawn from the vein, activate the shield by pressing it against any firm surface so that it swings over the needle. Because the shield is incorporated into the holder, the holder and needle assembly are discarded as one unit providing end-to-end needle protection. The device accommodates one-handed activation, an essential feature of an effective sharps injury protection device.

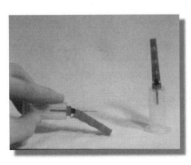

Portex Needle-Pro® (Sims Portex, Inc., Crystal Lake, IL)

Saf-T Clik®

The Saf-T Clik (MPS Acacia, Brea, CA) single-use tube holder has an inner sleeve that retracts the needle into the holder after the needle is removed from the patient's vein. To activate, the outer sleeve is extended over the needle, permanently locking and concealing the needle within. The concealed needle and holder are then discarded as one unit.

Saf-T Holder®

The Saf-T Holder (MPS Acacia, Brea, CA) is a modified tube holder that facilitates tube filling directly from vascular access devices. The holder incorporates a male luer that connects to vascular access systems such as needleless valves. Once in place, collection tubes are inserted into the holder and filled as they would be with conventional tube holders in venipunctures. After use, the single-use the holder is discarded into a sharps container.

Safety Needles

Products in this class allow for concealment or blunting of the contaminated sharp. They are activated either before or after removing the needle from the vein and are intended to reduce the healthcare worker's exposure to the sharp.

Punctur-Gard®

The Punctur-Gard (Bio-Plexus®, Vernon, CT) is a self-blunting needle that enters the vein sharp and and is made safe while still in the patient's vein, minimizing the user's exposure to the contaminated sharp. It has been reported by the CDC that use of this device can reduce the rate of accidental needlesticks by 76%.[6] The device is a two-part needle: the outer sharp to access the vein, and the inner blunt cannula to make the needle safe. The inner blunt cannula is recessed behind the sharp tip of the outer needle when the vein is accessed. When the blood collection procedure is complete, but before the

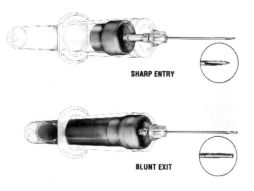

SHARP ENTRY

BLUNT EXIT

Punctur-Gard®
(Photo courtesy of Bio-Plexus, Vernon, CT)

needle is removed from the patient, the blunt cannula is advanced past the sharp tip. The safety feature is activated either by advancing the blood collection tube into the Punctur-Guard® standard holder or Drop-It® Holder, or by turning the dial on the Punctur-Guard Revolution™ Holder. The blunted needle is then discarded into a sharps container as usual. Because the contaminated sharp is blunted before it leaves the vein, the healthcare worker's risk of exposure to the contaminated sharp is minimized.

ECLIPSE™

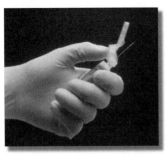

ECLIPSE™ (Photo courtesy of BD, Franklin Lakes, NJ)

The Eclipse, (BD, Franklin Lakes, NJ) employs a hinged sheath that is engaged over the needle, permanently covering it after use. To activate the safety feature, the collector pushes a plastic hinged sheath (referred to by the company as a "safety shield") over the contaminated sharp until an audible click is heard. Once concealed, the sharp is permanently sheathed and can be discarded into an approved sharps container. The Eclipse allows for immediate one-handed activation, an essential feature of an effective sharps injury protection device. It can be threaded onto conventional tube holders or with BD's Pronto® one-handed needle release tube holders.

Laser Skin Perforation Devices

Laser technology has been applied to devices that perforate the skin for near-painless capillary punctures These devices direct a pulse of light energy onto the skin vaporizing it 1-2 mm into the capillary bed, yielding blood in quantities sufficient for most bedside testing. Instead of the sharp pain associated with traditional lancets, patients feel a sensation similar to mild heat or pressure. Because such devices negate the use of lancets for tests that require small quantities of blood, they eliminate the risk of accidental needlesticks during capillary punctures. Wounds generated by this technology heal faster than those produced by lancets.[13] Laser skin perforation devices are not recommended in areas where oxygen is in use.

LASETTE™

The Lasette™ (Cell Robotics International, Inc., Albuquerque, NM) is a laser skin perforator that can be adjusted to yield volumes from one to two drops of blood (sufficient for most for bedside testing systems) to 100-200 microliters (for expanded laboratory testing). According to the company, the Lasette is the first medical laser device cleared by the FDA for use in the home, making it particularly beneficial to diabetic patients for self-testing.

LASER LANCET®

The Laser Lancet (Transmedica, Little Rock, AR) is a battery-operated laser emitting device intended for the perforation of skin to collect capillary blood specimens. The device directs a pulse of light energy onto the skin vaporizing it to 1-2 mm into the capillary bed. The amount of blood that penetration to this depth yields (about 100 microliters) is sufficient for most tests done at the bedside.

Plastic Collection Tubes

Glass blood tube pose a risk to healthcare professionals who handle blood specimens should they crack or break during collection, handling or transportation. Because there is a great deal of concern over the risk that glass poses to healthcare workers who handle specimens, tube manufacturers are offering plastic alternatives that significantly reduce the risk of exposure to bloodborne pathogens. Two companies have a complete line of plastic tubes while two others offer plastic versions of some of their products. Greiner Vacuette (Monroe, NC) and Sarstedt (Newton, NC) both manufacture a

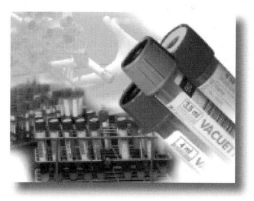

Greiner's (Monroe, NC) Vacuette® line of plastic collection tubes.

complete line of plastic blood specimen collection tubes exclusively. Greiner tubes can be used for conventional draws using tube holders and syringes whereas Sarstedt's line of S-Monovette® tubes are designed to be used with their dedicated blood collection needles.

Kendall's (Mansfield, MA) Corvac™ gel separator tubes are only available in plastic and BD (Franklin Lakes, NJ) offers plastic versions for most of their product line.

References

1 Latex Sensitivity: Clinical and Legal Issues. *The Risk Management Reporter.* ECRI. 16(4), Plymouth Meeting, PA. August 1977.

2 National Committee for Clinical Laboratory Standards (NCCLS): *Protection of Laboratory Workers from Instrument Biohazards and Infectious Disease Transmitted by Blood, Body Fluids, and Tissue.* Approved Guideline M29-A, Villanova, PA: December 1997.

3 Carlsen W, Holding R. Epidemic ravages caregivers; Thousands die from diseases contracted through needle sticks. *San Francisco Chronicle.* April 12, 1998.

4 Pallatroni L. Needlesticks: Who pays the price when costs are cut on safety? *MLO.* 1998;30(7):30.

5 Kearsly S. High profits—at what cost? *San Francisco Chronicle.* April 14, 1998.

6 Centers for Disease Control and Prevention. Evaluation of safety devices for pre-venting percutaneous injuries among health-care workers during phlebotomy procedures. *MMWR Morb Mortal Wkly Rep.* 1997;46(2):21-25.

7 Carlsen W, Holding R. Safety designs proposed but not produced. *San Francisco Chronicle.* April 12, 1998.

8 US Department of Labor and Occupational Safety and Health Administration (OSHA). Occupational exposure to bloodborne pathogens; final rule (29 CFR 1910.1030). *Federal Register.*1991;Dec 6:64004-64182.

9 Holding R, Carlsen W. Watchdogs fail health workers. *San Francisco Chronicle.* April 12, 1998. Available at http://www.sfgate.com. Accessed June 8, 1998.

10 Jagger, J. Rates of needlestick injury caused by various devices in a university hospital. N Engl J Med. 1988;319(5):284-288.

11 Statement by Secretary of Labor Alexis M. Herman on preventing needlestick injuries, May 20,1999. Available at http://osha.gov/media/statements/ndlstmt052099.html. Accessed May 21, 1999.

12 Needlestick prevention device selection guide. *Health Devices.* ECRI. Plymouth Meeting, PA. 2000.

13 Latshaw, J Laser takes the sting out of phlebotomy. *Adv Med Lab Professionals.* December 1, 1997.

Appendices

Appendix I
The Effects of Preanalytical Errors on Specimen Results

Error: Patient misidentification.

Result: Missed or erroneous diagnosis, general patient mismanagement, death.

Guideline: Acceptable means of identification consists of asking lucid patients to state their name and comparing their reply to the order requisitions and arm bracelet, which must be attached to the patient. If the patient cannot give a verbal response, a caregiver should identify the patient (document the name of the verifier) and the identity compared with the order requisition and arm bracelet.

Error: Incorrect order of draw.

Result: Falsely elevated potassium levels, spurious CBC results, contaminated blood cultures and erroneous coagulation results from cross-contamination of additives.

Guideline: Follow the correct order of draw when filling all blood tubes (see Chapter 3).

Error: Delays in processing.

Result: Decay of analyte. Inaccurate results that lead to misdiagnosis, over- or undermedication, patient mismanagement.

Guideline: Lavender-top tubes—for CBCs, results stable for 24 hours at refrigerated temperatures. For sed rates, results are stable for only 12 hours at refrigerated temperatures (4 hours unrefrigerated).

Blue-top tubes—PTT reliable for only 4 hours after collection, regardless of storage condition.

Red-top tubes—Refrigeration of red-top tubes without centrifugation or separation is disastrous to many analytes (see table below). Separate serum from cells within 2 hours unless evidence exists that longer contact times do not contribute to the inaccuracy of the result.

Effects of Serum/Cell Contact During Delays in Testing

Increase	Decrease
Potassium	Glucose
Phosphorous	Folate
Creatinine	Ionized calcium
B-12	CO_2
ALT	
AST	
Ammonia	
LDH	

Error: Collecting patient after a prolonged fast (>14 hours).
Result: Increases and decreases for the following tests:

Increase	**Decrease**
Amino acids	Glucose
Bilirubin	HDL cholesterol
Fatty acids	Insulin
Glucagon	LDH
Growth hormone	T3
Ketones	
Lactate	
Triglycerides	

Guideline: Avoid collecting patients who have fasted longer than 14 hours. If not possible, document the excessive fast for accurate interpretation of the results.

Error: Inappropriate coordination of collection time with time of medication dosage.
Result: Patient appears over- or under-medicated. Can result in unnecessary or life-threatening changes in dosage.
Guideline: Draw tests for therapeutic drug levels according to the drug's pharmacokinetics—ie, when the drug should be fully absorbed and at therapeutic levels—unless otherwise instructed by the physician.

Error: Inappropriate collection times for levels that vary according to biological rhythms.
Result: Misinterpretation of the following results:

Analytes that Vary According to Biological Rythms

Adrenocorticotropin	FSH	Triglycerides
Aldosterone	Growth hormone	TSH
Bilirubin	Luteinizing hormone	Uric Acid
BUN	Prolactin	
Catecholamines	Progesterone	
Cortisol	Testosterone	

Guideline: Most test results are compared against normal ranges established on early-morning collections. Collect levels that demonstrate diurnal variation in the morning, if possible. If not possible, ensure that time of collection is well-documented to facilitate accurate interpretation of the result.

Error: Collecting specimen immediately after patient has exercised.

Result: Increases in white blood cell count, AST, creatinine, bilirubin, uric acid, CK, cortisol, LD, ACTH, HDL, and the percentage of neutrophils in a CBC.

Guideline: Wait at least 1 hour after a rigorous exercise before drawing. If not possible, make a notation in the records to facilitate an accurate interpretation of the results.

Error: Leaving the tourniquet on longer than 1 minute before accessing vein.

Result: Elevated levels of potassium, total protein, calcium, bilirubin, ALT, AST, cholesterol, triglycerides, albumin, hemoglobin, and cell counts.

Guideline: Do not leave the tourniquet on for more than 1 minute before you access vein. Release tourniquet immediately after vein is accessed.

Error: Incomplete sterilization of site for blood culture collection.

Result: Contaminated blood culture. Possible extended stay and unnecessary antibiotics.

Guideline: Prepare the site according to recommended procedure (see Chapter 4).

Error: Not allowing cleansing solution to dry before puncture.

Result: If alcohol used to cleanse the site is not dried before the puncture it will alter glucose, potassium, phosphorous, and uric acid results and hemolyze the specimen. If an iodine or povidone solution used to cleanse the site is not dried before the puncture it will cause an increase in phosphorous, uric acid, and potassium.

Guideline: Allow thorough drying of the cleansing agent before puncturing site.

Error: Excessive probing, excessive pulling pressure on syringe plunger, or needle is not completely within the vein.

Result: Hemolysis that results in elevated levels of potassium, LDH, AST, ALT, phosphorous, magnesium, and ammonia; decreased levels of RBC, hemoglobin, and hematocrit; and a dilutional effect on all other analytes.

Guideline: Use gentle pulling pressure on syringe plunger or slightly relocate needle.

Error: Rimming clots clinging to inside of collection tube.

Result: Hemolysis; exposes the laboratorian to potential bloodborne pathogens.

Guideline: Stand specimens upright while clotting and allow 30 minutes before centrifugation.

Error: Anticoagulated specimen not inverted immediately after collection.

Result: Clotted specimen. If detectable, specimen will be rejected by laboratory. If not detectable, cell counts will be inaccurate.

Guideline: Invert all tubes with additives 5 to 10 times immediately after collection.

Error: Underfilling tubes with anticoagulants.

Result: Blue-top tubes—Inaccurate protime results.

Lavender-top tubes—Excessive anticoagulation, red cell shrinkage, falsely lower hematocrit and CBC indices.

Guideline: Fill all tubes with additives at least 75% of their full volume. Fill all blue-top tubes to 90% of their full volume.

Error: Inappropriate use of gel-type serum separator tubes.

Result: Falsely high or low therapeutic drug levels (TDMs), progesterone, tricyclic antidepressants. Also interferes with blood bank testing.

Guideline: Some tubes may be acceptable for some TDMs. Follow the tube manufacturer's guidelines on affected analytes. For other analytes, store separated serum on gel for 24 hours at refrigerated temperatures. Do not use for progesterone, tricyclic antidepressants, or blood bank specimens.

Error: Wrong tube.

Result: Grossly inaccurate results.

Guideline: Green-top tubes—Do not use green-top tubes containing lithium heparin for lithium levels. Use green tops with sodium heparin (tubes look identical).

Blue-top tubes—Do not use the blue-top tubes specifically designated for FDPs ("fibrin-split products" or "fibrin degradation" products) when collecting for PT, PTT, or factor assays. (Both tubes may have same color of stopper but have different additives and fill volumes.)

Error: Tests for bilirubin exposed to light.

Result: Result will be 50% lower after 1 hour of exposure to light.

Guideline: Collect specimens for bilirubin in amber, light-blocking tube, and/or enclose tube in light-tight transport container or wrap in aluminum foil immediately after collection.

Error: Blood gas specimens collected in plastic syringes not tested in 30 minutes.

Result: Gases migrate through plastic syringe barrel, altering concentrations in the arterial specimen.

Guideline: Transport all specimens to the testing facility within 30 minutes. If longer delays are unavoidable, collect the specimen in a glass syringe or transfer specimen into a heparinized glass blood collection tube (green top) and transport on ice.

Appendix II
Phlebotomy Resources

AIDS Exposure Hotline
Provides information to healthcare workers who have been exposed and to infection control officers who are managing exposures and exposure control plans. 1 (888) 448-4911.

Center for Phlebotomy Education
Provides phlebotomy conferences, workshops, seminars, teleconferences, books, videos, and other educational materials to healthcare professionals and facilities. Contact: Center for Phlebotomy Education, PO Box 161, Ramsey, IN 47166. Phone: (812) 633-4636; fax 812-633-2346; e-mail: phlebotomy@phlebotomy.com; Web site: http://www.phlebotomy.com.

CDC National AIDS Hotline: (800) 342-2437

COLA
A national healthcare accrediting organization. Provides comprehensive text and internet-based educational material on OSHA's Bloodborne Pathogen Standard as well as a full range of laboratory and medical practice issues. Contact: COLA, 9881 Broken Land Parkway, Suite 200, Columbia, MD 21046. Phone (800) 981-9883. Web site: http://www.cola.org.

College of American Pathologists (CAP)
Sets standards of performance for clinical laboratories through manuals, educational materials, proficiency examinations, and inspections. Contact: CAP, 325 Waukegan Rd, Northfield, IL 60093. Phone: (703) 446-8800; Web site: http://www.cap.org.

ECRI
A nonprofit health research agency. Publishes *Health Devices* monthly and other publications periodically. 5200 Butler Pike, Plymouth Meeting, PA 19462-1298; Phone: (610) 825-6000; Web site: http://www.ecri.org.

Exposure Prevention Information Network (EPINet)
Distributes software for tracking and reporting exposures. Phone: (770) 469-4098; Web site: http://www.med.virginia.edu/epinet/home.html.

Healthcare Worker Safety Project
Publishes *Advances in Exposure Prevention* and collects and distributes data on safety devices and needlestick injuries. Phone: (804) 924-5159; Web site: http://www.med.virginia.edu/medcntr/centers/epinet/subpage3.html.

Joint Commission on Accreditation of Healthcare Organizations (JCAHO)
Sets standards of performance for healthcare facilities through manuals, educational materials, and inspections. Contact: JCAHO, One Renaissance Blvd, Oakbrook Terrace, IL 60181. Phone: (630) 792-5000; Web site: http://www.jcaho.org.

National Committee for Clinical Laboratory Standards, (NCCLS)
Establishes and maintains standards of performance for laboratory procedures. Offers membership, published standards in printed and video (VHS) format, and software for healthcare facilities. Discounts available for member purchase. Contact: NCCLS, 940 W Valley Rd, Suite 1400, Wayne, PA 19087-1898. Phone: (610) 688-0100; Web site: http://www.nccls.org.

Occupational Safety and Health Administration (OSHA)
Establishes and maintains standards of performance for companies in all industries to guarantee the safety and health of employees. Contact: OSHA Technical Support Office, US Department of Labor, 200 Constitution Avenue, Washington, DC 20210. Phone: (202) 693-2300; Web site: http://www.osha.gov.

Phlebotomy Etc.
Provides continuing education and custom workshops for phlebotomists and other laboratory and POL support personnel in California. Contact: Sheila Clover PBT(ASCP), Director, Phlebotomy Etc., PMB 249, 1145 Second Avenue, Suite A, Brentwood, CA, 94513. (925) 240-0770; Web site: http://www.phlebotomyetc.com.

Appendix III
Listed Products and their Manufacturers

A.N.D.™—Automatic Needle Disconnect containment system. Post Medical, PO Box 29863, Atlanta, GA 30359. (800) 876-8768; http://www.postmedical.com.

AutoDrop™—The Kendall® Co., 15 Hampshire St, Mansfield, MA 02048-1139. (800) 962-9888; http://www.kendallhq.com.

Cepti-Seal Blood Culture Prep Kit II®—Medi-Flex® Hospital Products, 8717 W 110th St., Suite 750, Overland Park, Kansas, 66210. (800) 523-0502; http://www.medi-flex.com.

Drop-it™—Bio-Plexus®, 129 Reservoir Rd, Vernon, CT 06066. (800) 223-0010; http://www.bio-plexus.com.

Eclipse™—BD, One Becton Dr, Franklin Lakes, NJ 07417. (888) 237-2762; http://www.bd.com.

EZ-Cleans Plus™—SafeTec of America, Inc., 1055 East Delavan, Buffalo, NY 14215. (800) 456-7077.

Laser Lancet®—TransMedica™, 323 Center Street, Suite 1100, Littlerock, AK 72201. (888) 711-2345; http://www.TransMedicainc.com.

Lasette®—Cell Robotics International, Inc, 2715 Broadbent Pkwy NE, Albuquerque, NM 87107. (505) 343-1131; http://www.cellrobotics.com.

Microtainer®—BD, One Becton Dr, Franklin Lakes, NJ 07417. (888) 237-2762; http://www.bd.com.

Mobile Draw Station™—MarketLab, Inc, 4282 Brockton SE, Kentwood, MI 49512. (800) 237-3604.

Needlyzer™—MedPro, 817 Winchester Rd, Suite 200, Lexington, KY 40505. (606) 225-5375; http://www.needlyzer.com.

Nics$_X$™—Bio Medical Disposal. 3690 Holcomb Bridge Rd, Norcross, GA 30092. (888) 393-9595; http://www.biodisposal.com.

Nicky™—Helena Laboratories P.O. Box. 752, Beaumont, TX 77704. (800) 231-5663; http://www.helena.com.

Persist™—BD, One Becton Dr, Franklin Lakes, NJ 07417. (888) 237-2762; http://www.bd.com.

Phlebotomagician's Pediatric Magic Kit—Center for Phlebotomy Education, PO Box 161, Ramsey, IN 47166. (812) 633-4636; http://www.phlebotomy.com.

Point-Lok™—Sims Portex, Inc, 10 Bowman Dr, PO Box 724, Keene, NH 03431. (800) 258-5361; http://www.portexusa.com.

Pronto™—BD, One Becton Dr, Franklin Lakes, NJ 07417. (888) 237-2762; http://www.bd.com.

Punctur-Guard®—Bio-Plexus, 129 Reservoir Rd, Vernon, CT 06066. (800) 223-0010; http://www.bio-plexus.com.

QuickHeel™—BD, One Becton Dr, Franklin Lakes, NJ 07417. (888) 237-2762; http://www.bd.com.

Saf-T Clik®—MPS Acacia, 499 Nibus Street, Brea, CA 92821. (800) 299-4849; http://www.mpsacacia.com.

Saf-T Holder®—MPS Acacia, 499 Nibus Street, Brea, CA 92821. (800) 299-4849; http://www.mpsacacia.com.

Sharpx™—Bio Medical Disposal. 3690 Holcomb Bridge Rd, Norcross, GA 30092. (888) 393-9595; http://www.biodisposal.com.

Tenderfoot®—International Technidyne Corp., 87 Olsen Ave, Edison, NJ 08820. (800) 631-5945; http://www.itcmed.com.

Vacuette®—Greiner Vacuette North America, 260 Gateway Drive, Suite 17A, P.O. Box 943, Bel Air, Maryland 21024. (888) 286-3883; http://www.vacuette.com.

VanishPoint®—Retractable Technologies, 622 S Mill St, Lewisville, Texas 75057-4632. (888) 703-1010; http://www.vanishpoint.com.

Venipuncture Needle-Pro®—Sims Portex, Inc, 10 Bowman Dr, PO Box 724, Keene, NH 03431. (800) 258-5361; http://www.portexusa.com.

Appendix IV
Educational Resources

Part 1
Instructional Videos

ASCP Press
American Society of Clinical Pathologists
2100 West Harrison St
Chicago, IL 60612
Phone: (312) 738-1336
Web address: http://www.ascp.org

TITLE: *Blood Collection: The Difficult Draw*
   Not all patients have accessible veins. Not all patients are cooperative. This video discusses how to overcome physical, emotional and medical obstacles that make venipunctures difficult. Also discusses alternatives to antecubital punctures. Approximate running time: 25 minutes.

TITLE: *Blood Specimen: Special Procedures*
   This video discusses special procedures such as bleeding times, glucose tolerance tests, specimens for blood bank testing, special transport considerations, etc. Approximate running time: 22 minutes.

TITLE: *Blood Specimen: The Pediatric Patient*
   Techniques for collecting blood specimens from children and infants is discussed in this video including tips on calming fears and minimizing anxiety. Approximate running time: 20 minutes.

TITLE: *Blood Specimen: The Routine Venipuncture*
   This video discusses basic phlebotomy techniques. Sections include technique, equipment, safety, specimen labeling and handling. Approximate running time: 22 minutes.

BD Media Center
1 Becton Dr
Franklin Lakes, NJ 07417
Phone: (800) 255-6334
Fax: (201) 847-4862
Web address: http://www.bd.com

TITLE: *Modern Blood Collection Techniques*
Gives an overview of venipuncture using safe blood collection procedures and safe protective equipment. Approximate running time: 29 min.

TITLE: *Modern Blood Collection Techniques for Nurses*
Same as "Modern Blood Collection Techniques," but with a special introduction for nurses. Approximate running time: 33 min.

TITLE: *Blood Specimen Collection: Trouble-Shooting and Helpful Hints*
Identifies techniques to avoid blood collection problems and increase the quality of blood specimens. Approximate running time: 21 min.

TITLE: *Blood Specimen Transportation and Handling*
Focuses on proper handling of specimens collected at a location other than the hospital or reference lab, and the protection of healthcare workers and patients. Approximate running time: 8 min.

TITLE: *Blood Specimen Collection: Microcollection Techniques, Volume 4*
Integrates techniques, new collection devices, safety issues and patient care with procedures involving small amounts of blood.
Approximate running time: 14 minutes.

Center for Phlebotomy Education
P.O. Box 161
Ramsey, IN 47166
Phone: (812) 633-4636
Fax: (812) 633-2346
e-mail: phlebotomy@phlebotomy.com
Web site: http://www.phlebotomy.com

TITLE: *A Higher Standard*
> Lynda Arnold, a 26-year old registered nurse, suffered an accidental needlestick in 1992. Six months later she tested positive for HIV. This is her story. Ms. Arnold discusses the events that led to her accident and explores the personal implications and preventive issues surrounding accidental needlesticks. Experts in infection control and needlestick safety also discuss prevention and exposure issues. Produced by: National Campaign for Healthcare Worker Safety. Approximate running time: 40 minutes.

National Committee for Clinical Laboratory Standards (NCCLS)
940 West Valley Rd
Suite 1400
Wayne, PA 19087-1898
Phone: (610) 688-0100
Web address: http://www.nccls.org

TITLE: *Bedside Blood Glucose Testing: A Team Approach*
> This video is designed for nurses, administrators, and laboratorians and presents a team strategy for planning and developing a cohesive bedside blood glucose testing program. It includes recommendations for quality control, test perform-ance, and quality assurance. Sections on specimen collection, trouble-shooting and staff training are included. The NCCLS approved guideline is included with this video. Approximate running time: 18 minutes.

TITLE: *Quality Venipuncture: The Key to Accurate Results.*
> This video provides details on obtaining the highest quality blood specimen for laboratory testing with emphasis on the puncture procedure, safety, labeling and handling specimens. A printed copy of the NCCLS standard for venipunctures is included. Approximate running time: 25 minutes.

TITLE: *Quality Microcollection*
> This video illustrates how to obtain the highest quality skin punctrure specimen for laboratory testing. Sections include safety, advantages of performing skin punctures, supplies, the skin puncture procedure itself, handling, and labeling. A printed copy of the NCCLS standard for skin punctures is included. Approximate running time: 18 minutes.

Part 2
Phlebotomy Training Arms

Ambu, Inc.
611 N. Hammonds Ferry Rd
Linthicum, Maryland 21090
Phone: (800) 262-8462
Fax: (800) 262-8673
Web address: http://www.ambuusa.com

Armstrong Medical
575 Knightsbridge Pkwy
P.O. Box 700
Lincolnshire, IL 60069-0700
Phone: (800) 323-4220
Fax: (847) 913-0138
Web address: http://www.armstrongmedical.com

MarketLab
4282 Brockton
Kentwood, MI 49512
Phone: (800) 237-3604
Fax: (616) 656-2475

Medical Plastics Laboratory, Inc (MPL)
P.O. Box 38
226 F.M. 116 SO
Industrial Air Park
Gatesville, Texas, 76528
Phone: (800) 433-5539
Web address: http://www.medicalplastics.com

Venatech, Inc.
8475 Shadow Court
Coral Springs, FL 33021
Phone: (877) 904-9907
Fax: (954) 796-1611

Part 3
Phlebotomy Certification Study Guides

ASCP Press
American Society of Clinical Pathologists
2100 West Harrison St
Chicago, IL 60612
(312) 738-1336
Web address: http://www.ascp.org

TITLE: *Phlebotomy Review Guide*
　　　Susan E. Phelan
　　　Paperback, 1998

Appleton & Lange
Prentice Hall
One Lake St
Upper Saddle River, NJ 07458
Phone: (201) 236-3281
Fax: (201) 236-3290

TITLE: *Phlebotomy/Blood Collection*
　　　Kathleen Becan-McBride, Diana Garza
　　　400 questions, with disk.
　　　Softbound, 1998.

F A Davis & Company
1915 Arch St
Philadelphia, PA 19103
Phone: (800) 523-4049
Fax: (215) 568-5065
E-mail: info@fadavis.com

TITLE:*Phlebotomy Workbook for the Multiskilled Healthcare Professional*
　　　Susan King Strasinger, Marjorie A. Di Lorenzo
　　　Paperback, 1995

Lippincott, Williams & Wilkins
351 West Camden St
Baltimore, MD 21201
Phone: (800) 326-1685

TITLE: *Phlebotomy Exam Review*
           Ruth E. McCall, Cathee M. Tankersley
           Paperback and disk, 1996

Parthenon Pub Group
One Blue Hill Plaza
PO Box 1564, Pearl River
New York, NY 10965
Tel: (845) 735-9363
Toll Free: (800) 735-4744
Fax: (845) 735-1385
E-mail: usa@parthpub.com

TITLE: *Review Questions for Phlebotomy Examination*
           S.A. Taylor
           Paperback, 2000

Prentice Hall
One Lake St.
Upper Saddle River, NJ 07458
Phone: (201) 236-3281
Fax: (201) 236-3290

TITLE: *Phlebotomist Test Preparation*
           Cynthia M. Reed
           Textbook binding, 1995

Part 4
Web-Based Phlebotomy Tutorials

Virtual Phlebotomy—A dynamic phlebotomy tutorial from the University of Maryland at Baltimore School of Nursing. http://parsons.umaryland.edu/~vguy/phleb.htm.

Phlebotomy Overview—a comprehensive tutorial on blood collection procedures provided by the Syracuse University of New York's Upstate Medical University.
http://www.upstate.edu/phlebotomy

Web Path—a mini tutorial on venipunctures and capillary punctures. Includes many illustrations.
http://www-medlib.med.utah.edu/WebPath/TUTORIAL/PHLEB/PHLEB.html

Pre-Analytical Factors Affecting Laboratory Results—Part of the "Virtual Hopsital" series from the University of Iowa. Contains instructions on venipunctures, using tube holders, syringes and winged infusion sets, fingersticks and heelsticks. Participants have access to a practice test and evaluation form.
http://www.vh.org/Providers/CME/CLIA/Phlebotomy/Phlebotomy.html

Part 5
Training Software

Lippincott, Williams & Wilkins
351 West Camden St
Baltimore, MD 21201
Phone: (800) 326-1685

Phlebotomy Tutor—An interactive multimedia program with videoclips of proper phlebotomy procedures, three-dimensional animation demonstrating common errors, and a final exam to assess competency. Developed by the University of Washington Department of Laboratory Medicine.

Shiesl Corporation
1414 York Hill Road
Lincoln, VT 05443-8802
(802) 453-6196

Medicomp Module for Phlebotomy—Phlebotomy examination consisting of 100 phlebotomy questions with immediate feedback for wrong answers.

Part 6
National Phlebotomy Seminars,
Conferences and Workshops

Center for Phlebotomy Education
P.O. Box 161
Ramsey, IN 47166
812-633-4636
Web site: http://www.phlebotomy.com
E-mail: phlebotomy@phlebotomy.com

Conducts customized on-site in-services and workshops by invitation. Develops and presents phlebotomy seminars, conferences, and workshops nationwide. Approved provider of continuing education credits through the ASCLS P.A.C.E. program, Florida Board of Medical Laboratory Personnel, Florida Board of Nursing, and California Board of Registered Nursing. Also produces educational material and provides resources for all healthcare professionals who perform, supervise or teach phlebotomy.

National Laboratory Training Network
2121 W. Taylor Street
Chicago, IL 60612
(800) 536-6586
Web site: http://www.phppo.cdc.gov/dls/nltn/default.asp

Offers phlebotomy seminars, conference, and workshops nationwide. Also provides distance-based learning programs. Provides continuing education credit according to the criteria of the International Association for Continuing Education and Training.

Appendix V
Phlebotomy-Related Web Sites

The Drawing Room—http://clubs.yahoo.com/clubs/thedrawingroom

Hepatitis On the Web—A resource for information on hepatitis [needs research] Web site: www.hepnet.com

Phlebotomy Library of Links—a nice compilation of tutorials and links to phlebotomy organizations, publications, vendors, regulatory agencies, etc compiled by the Health Science Center of Syracuse.
Web address: http://upstate.edu.80/phlebotomy/pages/library/organizations.htm

Phlebotomy Etc.—an educational organization that posts a monthly phlebotomy newsletter containing topical news and issues in phlebotomy.
Web address: http://www.phlebotomyetc.com

Phlebotomy Today—Online phlebotomy newsletter covering news items, tips on technique, and new products. Includes the "Phlebotomy Tip of the Month" designed to be printed and posted in collection areas.
Web address: http://www.phlebotomy.com

Southern California Phlebotomy Training—offers a comprehensive list of phlebotomy schools, certifying agencies, continuing education and links to other phlebotomy sites. Also offers phlebotomy supplies, education materials and mechanical training aids.
Web address: http://www.scpt.com

UCLA Library Resource—This unique site offers a history of bloodletting including illustrations on ancient anatomy and bloodletting instruments.
Web address:
http://www.library.ucla.edu/libraries/biomed/his/blood/blood1.htm

Appendix VI
Phlebotomy Certification Organizations

American Certification Agency (ACA)
P.O. Box 58
Osceola, IN 46561
Phone: (219) 277-4538
Web address: http://www.acacert.com

Requirements to take written and practical test:
high school diploma and
1) One year of experience OR
2) Successful completion of an approved phlebotomy program.

Continuing education is required to renew certification every 2 years.

American Medical Technologists (AMT)
710 Higgins Road
Parkridge, IL 60068-5765
Phone: (847)823-5169
Web address: http://www.amt1.com

Requirements to take written exam:
High school diploma or equivalent and

1) Graduation from a phlebotomy course in a school or program accredited by the Accrediting Bureau of Health Education Schools (ABHES) plus completion of a minimum of 50 venipunctures and 25 finger/heel sticks, OR
2) Graduation from an acceptable program in an institution accredited by an agency recognized by the United States Departments of Education or the Commission on the Recognition of Postsecondary Accreditation (COPRA) plus completion of at least 50 venipunctures and 25 finger/heel sticks, OR
3) Successful completion of an acceptable phlebotomy training program, which includes at least 120 hours of clinical practica and a minimum of 50 venipunctures and 25 finger/heelsticks, OR
4) Completion of at least 1040 hours of acceptable work experience as a phlebotomy technician within the past three years; this is to include at least 50 venipunctures, 25 skin punctures, specimen processing, communication skills, and clerical duties.

American Medical Technologists (AMT) (cont.)

Examination waived if applicant:

1) Has passed a phlebotomist examination for the purpose of state licensure or

2) Holds other phlebotomy certification obtained by examination and are determined by the Board to have met the AMT training and experience requirements.

Continuing education not required to remain certified.

American Society for Clinical Pathologists (ASCP)

2100 West Harrison St

Chicago, IL 60612

(312) 738-1336

Web address: http://www.ascp.org

Requirements to take written examination:

high school diploma (or equivalent) and

1) Completion of a National Accreditation Agency for Clinical Laboratory Science (NAA-CLS)-approved phlebotomy program within the last 5 years, OR

2) Completion of an acceptable formal structured phlebotomy program, which includes 120 clinical hours with a minimum performance of 100 successful venipunctures, 25 successful capillary punctures, observation of 5 arterial punctures, orientation in a full-service laboratory and 40 clock-hours of didactic training at a regionally-accredited college/university or laboratory within the last 5 years, OR

3) 1 year of full time experience as a phlebotomy technician in an accredited laboratory within the last 5 years, which included venipunctures, capillary punctures, observation of arterial punctures and orientation in a full-service laboratory, OR

4) Completion of an accredited allied health professional/occupational education with phlebotomy training including performance of a minimum of 100 successful venipunctures, 25 successful capillary punctures, observation of five arterial punctures and orientation in a full-service laboratory.

Continuing education not required to remain certified.

American Society of Phlebotomy Technicians (ASPT)

PO Box 1831
Hickory, NC 28603
Phone: (828) 294-0078
Web address: www.aspt.org

Requirements to take written and practical exam:
1) One year part time phlebotomy experience OR
2) Six months full time phlebotomy experience OR
3) Successful completion of an approved phlebotomy program including documentation
   of 100 successful venipunctures and 25 successful skin punctures.

Requirements for waiver from written and practical exam:
1) A letter from a health care professional attesting that part of the applicant's job is
   procuring blood specimens regularly.

Continuing education required to renew certification annually.

National Credentialing Agency (NCA)
PO Box 15945-289
Lenexa, KS 66285
(913) 438-5110 ext. 647
Web address: http://www.nca-info.org

Requirements to take written exam:
High school diploma and

1) Successful completion of an approved phlebotomy program that includes a clinical
   component in phlebotomy, OR
2) 1 year of full-time work experience including phlebotomy.

Continuing education is required to renew certification every three years.

National Center for Competency Testing (NCCT)
7007 College Blvd
Overland Park, KS 66211
Phone: (800) 875-4404
Web Address: http://ncctinc.com

Requirements to take written exam:
High school diploma or equivalent plus successful completion of an approved phlebotomy program.
Requirement for waiver from taking exam: documentation of at least one year of experience.

Continuing education required to renew certification annually.

National Healthcare Association (NHA)
194 Route 46
East Fairfield, NJ 07004
Phone: (800) 499-9092
Web address: www.nhainfo.com

Requirements to take written exam:
High school diploma or equivalent and

1) Successful completion of an approved phlebotomy program, OR
2) One year of phlebotomy experience.

Requirement for waiver from exam:
2 years of phlebotomy experience and completion of a home-study packet

Continuing education required for recertification every 2 years.

National Phlebotomy Association (NPA)
1901 Brightseat Rd
Landover, MD 20785
Phone: (301) 386-4200
Web address: http://www.scpt.com

Requirements to take written and practical exam:
Successful completion of an approved phlebotomy course.
Requirements for waiver from written and practical exams: At least 1 year of phlebotomy
    employment and submission of a Proficiency Evaluation Form to be completed by the
    applicant's employer. Also certifies phlebotomy instructors.

Continuing education required to renew certification annually.

Part 6
Audio Tapes

Provides audio tapes with slides on a variety of phlebotomy topics including:
  • Protecting Yourself From Phlebotomy-Related Lawsuits
  • Identifying and Eliminating Preanalytical Errors During Specimen Collection
  • Seizing Control of Blood Culture Contamination Rates
  • Needlestick Safety: Practices, Products and Legislative Updates

Programs consists of:
  • one 50-60 minute studio-recorded audiocassette
  • accompanying 35mm color slides
  • supplemental handout material
  • forms to complete and return for continuing education credit.

Center for Phlebotomy Education
P.O. Box 161
Ramsey, IN 47166
Phone: (812) 633-4636
Fax: (812) 633-2346
e-mail: phlebotomy@phlebotomy.com
Web site: http://www.phlebotomy.com

Appendix VII

The Ten Commandments of Phlebotomy

I

Thou shalt protect thyself from injury. Using gloves, needle disposal units, and proper technique can minimize your risk of becoming one of the estimated one million healthcare workers who will experience an accidental needle-stick this year. Thousands will contract some form of hepatitis. Fifty to sixty of them will acquire HIV.

II

Thou shalt identify thy patients. This means referring to an identifying bracelet affixed to the patient or asking the patient to state his or her name. When this is not possible, have the patient's caregiver identify the patient and document the person who verified it for you. No other methods are acceptable.

III

Thou shalt puncture the skin at about a fifteen degree angle. Most textbooks and standards agree on a fifteen to thirty degree angle of insertion. Injure a patient while puncturing at a greater angle and you will have a difficult time convincing the jury that you are immune from the standards.

IV

Thou shalt glorify the medial vein. The medial vein is the vein of choice for four reasons: 1) it's more stationary; 2) it hurts less; 3) it's usually closer to the surface of the skin; and 4) it isn't nestled amongst nerves or arteries. Keep the basilic vein as a last resort. Most nerve injuries and arterial nicks result from misguided punctures into this vein.

V

Thou shalt invert tubes with anticoagulants immediately after collection. A high percentage of blood specimens rejected by testing labs are due to clots in lavender- or blue-top tubes. A quick inversion after collection prevents a second puncture.

VI

Thou shalt attempt to collect specimens only from an acceptable site. Antecubital and hand veins are acceptable unless their use is precluded by intravenous infusions, injury, or mastectomy. Any other site should be approached with great trepidation. Should an injury occur, your puncture site had better be defensible in court.

VII

Thou shalt label specimens at the bedside. This means complete identification, not just temporary identifiers to help you when you find time to label them more completely later. Find time NOW! Patients have died as a result of mislabeled specimens.

VIII

Thou shalt stretch the skin at the puncture site. This accomplishes two functions: it anchors the vein and it minimizes the pain of the puncture. Your patients will thank you for considering their suffering.

IX

Thou shalt know when to quit. Not everyone can draw blood from every patient. Even those who elevate phlebotomy to an art form can have difficulty from time to time. After two failed attempts, one should seriously consider sending in someone else. It may be the answer to your patient's prayers.

X

Thou shalt treat all patients as if they were family. In a hospital, the only peace many patients experience is that which you bring them by your kind words, gentle technique, and your smile. Regardless of what you might think, you have been assigned to healthcare by a higher authority because of the comfort you can offer to the sick and injured. You haven't been employed; you've been ordained.

A four-color graphic poster of these proposed "commandments" is available from the Center for Phlebotomy Education at www.phlebotomy.com. See back pages for order information.

Appendix VIII

Bibliography

Becan-McBride K et al. *Health Question and Answer Review for Phlebotomy and Blood Collection.* Upper Saddle River, NJ. Prentice Hall; 2000.

Davis B. *Phlebotomy: A Client-Based Approach.* New York: Delmar Publishers; 1997.

Flynn J. *Procedures in Phlebotomy,* 2nd ed. Philadelphia, PA: W.B. Saunders Co.; 1999.

Fremgen B, Blume W. *Phlebotomy Basics.* Upper Saddle River, NJ. Prentice Hall; 2000.

Garza D, Becan-McBride K. *Phlebotomy Handbook: Blood Collection Essentials,* 5th ed. Norwalk, CT: Appleton & Lange; 1999.

Hoeltke, L. *The Complete Textbook of Phlebotomy.* New York: Delmar Publishers; 1999.

Hoeltke, L. *Phlebotomy: The Clinical Laboratory Manual Series.* New York: Delmar Publishers; 1995.

Kiechle FL, Chambers LM, Chiricosta FM, et al. *So You're Going to Collect a Blood Specimen,* 7th ed. College of American Pathologists (CAP), 325 Waukegan Rd, Northfield, IL 60093-2750, 1996.

Kovanda, B. *Phlebotomy Collection Procedures.* New York: Delmar Publishers; 1998.

McCall, R, Tankersley, C. *Phlebotomy Essentials,* 2nd ed. Philadelphia, PA: Lippincott-Raven Publishers; 1998.

National Committee for Clinical Laboratory Standards (NCCLS): *Procedures for the Collection of Diagnostic Blood Specimens by Skin Puncture,* Approved Standard H4-A4, Villanova, PA: NCCLS; 1999.

National Committee for Clinical Laboratory Standards (NCCLS). *Procedures for the Collection of Diagnostic Blood Specimens by Venipuncture.* Approved Standard H3-A4, Villanova, PA: NCCLS; 1998.

National Committee for Clinical Laboratory Standards (NCCLS). *Procedures for the Handling and Processing of Blood Specimens.* Approved Standard H18-A2,Villanova, PA: NCCLS; 1999.

National Committee for Clinical Laboratory Standards (NCCLS): *Protection of Laboratory Workers from Instrument Biohazards and Infectious Disease Transmitted by Blood, Body Fluids, and Tissue.* Approved Guideline, M29-A, Villanova, PA: NCCLS; December, 1997.

National Committee for Clinical Laboratory Standards. *Transport and Processing of Blood Specimens for Coagulation Testing and General Performance of Coagulation Assays.* Approved Standard H21-A3, Villanova, PA: NCCLS; 1998.

Pendergraph G, Pendergraph C. *Handbook of Phlebotomy and Patient Service Techniques.* 4th ed. Philadelphia, PA: Lippincott, Williams & Wilkins; 1998.

Phelan, S. *Phlebotomy Techniques: A Curriculum Guide.*Chicago, IL. ASCP Press; 1993

Phelan, S. *Phlebotomy Techniques: A Laboratory Workbook .*Chicago, IL. ASCP Press; 1993.

Southern California Phlebotomy Training (SCPT). *Preventing Needlesticks*. (SCPT, 23010 Lake Forest Dr, Suite 165, Laguna Hills, CA 92653.) (714) 362-1634. 1996.

US Department of Labor and Occupational Safety and Health Administration (OSHA). Occupational exposure to bloodborne pathogens; final rule (29 CFR 1910.1030). *Federal Register.*1991;Dec 6:64004-64182.

Index

V

W

The
⚔en Commandments of Phlebotomy
Poster

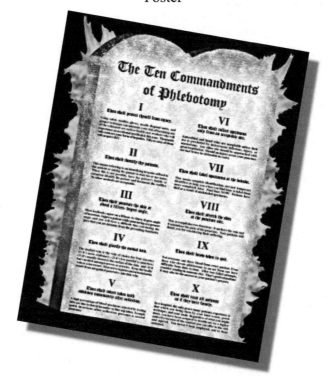

This 16x20 four-color poster from the Center for Phlebotomy Education serves as an eye-catching reminder to those collecting blood specimens in your facility to practice blood collection techniques that protect patients from injury, safeguard themselves from accidental needlesticks, produce uncompromised specimens, and demonstrate compassion for the patient. Some proposed "commandments" include:

⚔hou Shalt Protect Thyself From Injury

⚔hou Shalt Label Specimens at the Bedside

⚔hou Shalt Treat All Patients as if They Were Family

⚔hou Shalt Invert Tubes with Additives Immediately After Collection

When framed and displayed prominently in outpatient drawing areas, this poster also serves as visible evidence of your facility's ongoing commitment to quality patient care.

To Order the 𝔗𝔢𝔫 ℭ𝔬𝔪𝔪𝔞𝔫𝔡𝔪𝔢𝔫𝔱𝔰 𝔬𝔣 𝔓𝔥𝔩𝔢𝔟𝔬𝔱𝔬𝔪𝔶 Poster:

Fill out the form below and mail or fax to:
Center for Phlebotomy Education, P.O. Box 161, Ramsey, IN 47166
Fax: 812-633-2346
Please allow 2-4 weeks for delivery. Indiana facilities exempt from sales tax must include proof of exemption. Ten percent discount on orders of ten or more.

Shipping Address:

Addressee:_____

Facility Name:_____

Address:_____

City, State:_____ Zip:_____

QTY:	Price each	Subtotal
	$16.95	

5% Sales Tax (**Indiana Only**)

Shipping (up to ten posters to same address) | 3.50

Total

Method of Payment

☐ Check Enclosed   ☐ Visa   ☐ MasterCard   ☐ American Express

Credit Card Number_____ Expiration Date:_____

Name as it appears on card:_____

Signature:_____

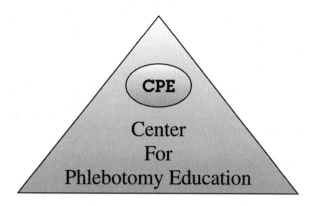

The Center for Phlebotomy Education

Mission Statement

To provide resources to the healthcare community that proper phlebotomy technique with emphasis on protecting healthcare workers and their patients from injury while obtaining high quality specimens for laboratory testing.

To provide comprehensive phlebotomy education to allied healthcare professionals through workshops, conference presentations, teleconferences, educational materials, and contributions to the literature.

To provide educational resources and products to phlebotomy educators.

The Center For Phlebotomy Education is founded to respond to the increased risk all healthcare workers assume when assigned phlebotomy responsibilities. It is the belief of the Center that those properly trained in venipuncture procedures are less likely to suffer accidental needlesticks from contaminated needles, less likely to injure patients, and more capable of providing testing labs with specimens free of variables introduced during collection and processing that alter results.

The Center achieves its mission by developing educational programs on all aspects of blood collection procedures and making them available by conducting:

- ➢ conferences nationwide
- ➢ customized in-services by invitation
- ➢ presentations at state, national and international meetings of healthcare organizations and associations
- ➢ Providing audio tapes and slides on selected phlebotomy topics,

In conjunction with *HealthStar Press*, the Center publishes and distributes printed and electronic resources such as:

- ➢ *Phlebotomy Today*---an online newsletter covering industry trends, phlebotomy tips (attractively designed to be printed and posted monthly!) and late-breaking legislative and regulatory events. View the newsletter at www.phlebotomy.com

- ➢ The *Ten Commandments of Phlebotomy* poster currently on display in hundreds of hospitals around the world.

- ➢ *Phlebotomy Resource Guide*---a comprehensive listing of educational resources including certification study guides, phlebotomy videos, textbooks, CD-ROM tutorials, certification agencies and their requirements, sources for training arms and other educational tools. (This is an expanded version of this book's appendices.)

Continuing Education Provider Information

For Laboratorians: The Center for Phlebotomy Education is approved as a provider of continuing education programs in the clinical laboratory sciences through the ASCLS P.A.C.E. program for all states including California. The Center is also an approved provider for the Florida Board of Clinical Laboratory Personnel.

For Nurses: The Center is approved by the California Board of Registered Nursing and the Florida Board of Nursing as a provider of continuing education credits for nurses. Other state nursing boards may have a reciprocal agreement to accept credits issued by out-of-state providers.

To schedule an in-service or workshop in your facility or for information on upcoming conferences in your area, visit our website at www.phlebotomy.com or contact us at:

Center for Phlebotomy Education
P.O. Box 161
Ramsey, IN 47166
812-633-4636 phone
812-633-2346 fax
E-mail: phlebotomy@phlebotomy.com

About the Authors

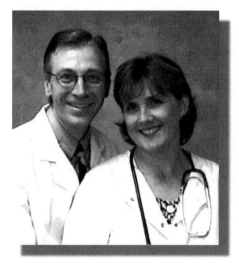

Dennis J. Ernst MT(ASCP) has been involved in phlebotomy for over 20 years as a medical technologist, educator and legal consultant. One of the most widely published authors on the subject of phlebotomy, Ernst is often recruited to speak at state and national healthcare conferences. As the Director of the Center for Phlebotomy Education, he conducts workshops, in-services and conferences on phlebotomy nationwide with the goal of protecting healthcare workers and their patients from injury while obtaining high quality specimens for laboratory testing. His credentials include:

➢ Phlebotomy instructor at the University of Louisville (Kentucky) School of Allied Health Sciences.
➢ Observing Member of the NCCLS Subcommittee on Blood Collection Procedures.
➢ Widely published author on phlebotomy for magazines including *Parents, Medical Laboratory Observer (MLO), Laboratory Medicine, RN, Journal of Healthcare Risk Management*, and others.
➢ Highly recruited speaker for nursing, laboratory, and allied health conferences nationwide.
➢ Retained by attorneys across the U.S. as an expert witness in phlebotomy liability cases.
➢ Nationally recognized phlebotomy authority.

Catherine Ernst, RN is a registered nurse with over 23 years of experience in acute and intensive care nursing, home care nursing, management and teaching. She currently serves as Nursing Liaison for the Center for Phlebotomy Education and works as a nurse educator in phlebotomy and IV insertion in an acute care hospital.